Organic (

Minister

Fuel for the Body

Your tools to optimum weight, radiant skin and vibrant health. Also helps you to enhance your libido!

LIVE HAPPY. BE PURE!

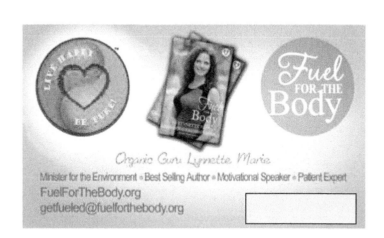

Organic Guru Lynnette Marie
Medicine Woman & Minister for the Environment

www.fuelforthebody.org
www.pureintegrityverified.com

Disclaimer:

All statements and protocols in this book are my own opinion and my own information based upon the research I have done.

Seek the advice from your natural practicing health care provider before making any life style changes.

***The statements in this book are not meant for treatment, cure or prevention of any disease or sickness and these statements have not been regulated by the FDA.

CREDITS

Book Cover: Jeff Stuchala, Howard Hoffman

Graphics: Jeff Stuchala
Chief Creative Officer
Personal Product Development, LLC
www.phreshproducts.com

Cover Picture: Roxana Ireland: Roxxe Photography
www.roxxephotography.com

Random Picture credits: Organic Consumers Association, Royalty Free pictures and compliments of sponsor's products, Lynnette's own pictures.

Endorsements:
Jordan S. Rubin Founder and CEO of Garden of Life and Beyond.Organic
www.beyondorganicinsider.com

Dr. Ramah J. Wagner; Chiropractor
www.doctorramah.com

Debra Clarke; Acupuncture Physician
Owner of the White Peacock Wellness Center

Selina DeLangre
Owner and CEO of Selina Naturally and Celtic Sea Salt
www.celticseasalt.com

Dr. Jenna Henderson
The Holistic Kidney
www.theholistic-kidney.com

Dr. Patrick Vickers
The Gerson Treatment Center
www.gersontreatment.com

Shan Stratton: CEO of Core Health Products
Consultant to major league sports teams
www.corehealthproducts.com

Howard Hoffman
CEO of Phresh Products
www.phreshproducts.com

Sally Malanga
CEO/Founder
Ecco Bella
www.eccobella.com

Tyler Ward
CEO/Founder
Giddy Organics
www.getgiddy.com

Laurye Natale
Director/Founder
America's Outstanding Mom
www.americasoutstandingmom.com

Robert Wright
Author of Killing Cancer NOT People
Founder of the American Anti-Cancer Institute
www.americanaci.org

Jeff Davis
CEO/Founder
Go Green America TV
www.gogreenamericatv.com

Liana Werner-Gray
CEO/Creator
The Earth Diet
www.theearthdiet.com

Glen B. Stewart
Globally acclaimed Author
Visions Of A Champion
www.ultrapro1.com

What Others Are Saying

"Lynnette Pate is a wonderful enlightening soul that is making a huge impact on the quality of our lives by creating opportunities for us to change the way we treat our foods and educates us to make healthier choices in life."

~ Zebulon Thomas
www.zebulonthomas.com
Author, Speaker & Life Coach

"Lynnette Pate's tireless dedication to educating the public on the importance of eating organic and non-gmo foods, as well as her relentless pursuit of exposing the corrupt forces within our society destroying our health through their modern food production mechanisms, should serve as an inspiration to anyone seeking to empower and better their lives through the use of pure and proper nutrition. I have a clinic where we are treating people for their advanced diseases; including terminal cancer. If my patients would have had the opportunity to be properly educated and inspired by people like Lynnette Pate BEFORE they got sick they would not be in the terrible predicament they are in when coming to my clinic. In this society of poisoned and altered foods, which are clearly causing a myriad of degenerative diseases, Lynnette's book plays an increasingly important role in educating people on the Truth. Thank you Lynnette for being a perpetual and relentless voice against the powers that continually try to destroy our lives and the lives of our children. Furthermore, your "Lynnette Doll" is going to be a wonderful inspiration

to young girls all around the country and will help to put them on a pure foundation by shaping the way they see their health and their bodies; a very powerful medium that is desperately needed in this deceptive world of manipulating our children's minds through corrupt advertising and marketing methods."

~ Dr. Patrick Vickers
Northern Baja Gerson Center
www.gersontreatment.com

"It has been a pleasure getting to know you and reading your book. Your passion and knowledge will certainly change the life of many people and I look forward to participating in your journey. Also, I feel honored to have shared the stage with you because TOGETHER we will make a difference".

~ Shan Stratton
CEO; Core Health Products
Consultant to Major league sports teams
www.corehealthproducts.com

"Go Green America TV and it's Host Jeff Davis "the Go Green Guy", are spreading the word on Healthy, Eco - Friendly, Green Living and we are so glad to have met and have the opportunity to work with Lynnette and the Fuel For the Body T.O.U.R. as she is a leader in spreading the message of Healthy Organic eating and Lifestyle".

~ Jeff Davis
AKA: The Go Green Guy
www.gogreenamericatv.com

7

"I found Lynnette Pate's breakthrough book "Fuel For The Body" to be a revitalizing and refreshing perspective on the growing Organic Movement. Most importantly, Lynnette provides the real world approach to incorporating life transforming organic meals and nutritional supplements in your lifestyle all without leaving one feeling like you are on a 'Weight Loss Diet'... We all intimately know how long 'That Painful Diet Approach' lasts...." "Lynnette Pate is an inspiring and a wealth of life transforming Organic Health knowledge, and she unleashes all her passion into sharing it in a rewarding, actionable way".

~ Glen B. Stewart Globally Acclaimed Author
"Visions Of A Champion"
www.ultrapro1.com

"The application of preventative medical principals in our lives can be defined as learning how to care for our whole selves, mind, body and spirit, followed by accepting responsibility of self-nurturing. The Pate Weigh uncovers the simple basics of the "how" and provides us tools needed to achieve self-empowerment".

~ Dr. Debra Clarke, Acupuncture Physician
The White Peacock Center, Lake Mary, FL

"Fuel for the Body" is an excellent resource for anyone who wants to shed pounds or improve overall health. Lynnette Pate's holistic plan includes sound guidelines that will not only steer the reader away from processed foods, but will explain why whole foods are healing for the body, soul and spirit. her nutritional background combined with a firm, no-nonsense approach about GMO foods and

pharmaceuticals are not the answer will truly inspire readers to choose preventative principles that can result in a life time of better health and nutrition. From choosing 3 "super food staples" to incorporating exercise into a daily routine. Fuel for the Body explores a better way to stave off cravings, prevent diseases and maintain an ideal weight."

~ Jordan S. Rubin: Founder of Garden of Life and Beyond Organic and NYT's best-selling author of 'The Maker's Diet'
www.beyondorganicinsider.com

"I used Organic Guru Lynnette Pate as a reference many times in TED book!!! :))) She is the WOMAN WARRIOR PIONEER freaking awesome human being who is demanding that GMO is on labels! and so much more :))) ♥ *people who are spreading health"!*

~ Liana Werner-Gray, Australian Actress
Author of The Earth Diet
www.theearthdiet.com

"Lynnette is one of those people who come into your life who makes you adopt their passion through the intrinsic motivation of actually wanting to be a part of what they are doing. Her drive and dedication to the green lifestyle is infectious as it is not something to envy but to imitate. Furthermore, she can be so generous with her time and knowledge that you forget you are even sitting with a true organic guru. As a green business owner, Lynnette has opened doors for me that I didn't even know previously existed. She is a spectacular and wonderful person to know even if you all you need is

9

simply a caring friend. If I had to describe her in one word it would be awesome or....Organic"!

~Tyler Ward; CEO of Giddy Organics
www.getgiddy.com

"Living an enlightened life starts with shedding pounds, toxins & limiting beliefs. The Pate Way is a clean way to begin the process of shedding. Lynnette's work speaks for itself. Don't be "weighed" down by unwanted toxins".

Dr. Ramah Wagner;
Author of 'The Health of Business'
www.healthofbusiness.com

"We at Ecco Bella applaud Lynnette Pate for her tireless efforts to educate the public on healthful, sustainable and cruelty   free   lifestyles. We are honored to have her as our ambassador and to be able to support her in her own mission to spread the word about healthy living. Whether riding her bike across the country or spreading the word through her book, Fuel For The   Body,   Lynnette   LIVES   it! Lynnette has been a long-time supporter of Ecco Bella's products and of our mission to provide natural, organic, gluten and paraben-free skin care and cosmetics to the conscientious consumer. Lynnette's tireless efforts are an inspiration to us all".

Sincerely,

Sally Malanga
Founder/ CEO Ecco Bella / New Earth Beauty
www.eccobella.com

"I am writing this letter to endorse Lynnette Marie Pate. My experience in these past 5 years with Lynnette Pate has been nothing less than delightful.

Lynnette is spending all of her time researching, and getting the word out about nutrition. She is the real deal. I give her the highest recommendation for being a representation of my Celtic Sea Salt® brand and the entire Selina Naturally line.

Our companies, Celtic Sea Salt® and Selina Naturally have been right behind Lynnette as she began her first journey tour across the nation in April of 2011. The respect and return of support she has given back to our companies has been well worth our investments in her. Lynnette is a true kindred spirit who truly seeks to help people heal their bodies and souls naturally. We will continue to support each of her endeavors in regards to the health world. She brings joy and harmony to our companies. We have our very own Lynnette Doll show cased in our corporate office.

Lynnette's book and tours are making a difference in the way the community is thinking about food. Lynnette is reaching hundreds of people that wouldn't hear of the truths in her book if she didn't reach out through her powers of tours.

Keep up the good work, one tour at a time".

Selina Delangre
CEO of Celtic Sea Salt® Brand since 1976 & Selina
Naturally www.celticseasalt.com

"Lynnette Pate is one of the most extraordinary women I have ever known! We met when she entered our competition for America's Outstanding Mom a couple years ago. After hearing her story about how she was able to cure her own son naturally of his debilitating disease, and of her crusade to educate the country on the benefits of living the much healthier lifestyle of organics via a bicycle, I realized that she was truly one of a kind. I could think of no one better to have as our Ambassador for America's Outstanding Mom than someone who makes it her personal mission to help every child live a happy and healthy life, and that person is Lynnette Pate, the Organic Guru"!

Laurye Natale
Founder and Director
America's Outstanding Mom
www.americasoutstandingmom.com

"I am very excited and honored to write this endorsement letter for Mrs. Lynnette Pate. My experience has been nothing less than wonderful.

Lynette's passion for helping people is inspiring. She works tirelessly to bring wellness and to educate the world by sharing and educating her mission. She is dedicated, hardworking, and a genuinely nice person that operates from her heart. Her enthusiasm for helping people live healthier lives is inspiring. Through her passion she enlightens the world with her knowledge of how to maintain health and achieve optimum wellness.

I am grateful to be a colleague and wish her all the luck in all of her future endeavors".

~ Howard Hoffman
CEO/Founder
Personal Health Product Development
www.phreshproducts.com

"One of the most studied and knowledgeable people about what fuels and heals the human body, it is highly likely that Lynnette Marie cares more about your health than you do. Her passion for wellness – and purity within that process – serves as a beacon for all who are searching for the real truth about what it takes to stay healthy and heal when you are not. At the International Wellness and Research Center (AACI), we are both proud and honored to have her as our Midwest Regional Ambassador and Product Integrity Advisory. Folks, listen closely to this woman – she knows whence she speaks".

~ Robert Wright, Director and Founder of the American Anti-Cancer Institute International Wellness & Research Center Author: "Killing Cancer – Not People"
www.americanaci.org

Dedication

I dedicate this book and the travels of our awesome T.O.U.R.s across the nation to my never wavering and loving Dad. Harold Hagar. He gave me the courage to keep pressing on. He gave me insight to what is going on in America. He helped me to understand truths and fictions. He gave me the stubborn gene to make me not take NO or YES for an answer. Without the intuition from my dad and the positive vibes he sent out, I would not be who I am today. He lived life to the very fullest and refused to let anything bring him down or make him unhappy. He always lived his life HAPPY! My father was tragically taken away from me the summer of 2013. He is and will be deeply missed. I will continue to take his energy to keep pressing on for truth, purity, health and happiness.

I LOVE YOU DAD!

*A special dedication will go in honor of my best friend; Grandma Ruby. She would have so enjoyed this book. I know she is with me today.

Table of Contents

Preface

What if I told you that you could live a life FREE of diseases, illnesses, sickness, obesity, free from weight struggle? What if I told you that you could have the weight of your dreams, the vibrant health you need, the glowing skin we all desire and even enhance your libido? Want to be FREE from Rx drugs, over the counter drugs and ailments? If you are tired of being tired, sick of being sick and need more stamina throughout the day. Or if you have been going in circles trying to find that 'perfect' diet to get you on the path to happiness, maybe you long to have radiant – glowing skin. Have you or your spouse been searching for that extra pick me up to naturally enhance your libido? Then this book is sure to get you on your way to better health, radiant skin and ultimate sex! You can have all that I have listed above. You can have the weight of your desire without counting calories, fat grams or points. You can have all this and never deprive yourself of yummy treats and eat what you want. Food (real food that is) is your key to success! You can also call me for a consultation on nutrition that will forever change the way you view food.

The biggest concerns I am hearing from my clients are:

a)   I can't do organic, it is too expensive.
b)   It's too time consuming and not convenient.

Well my answer to those questions is: What is your health worth to you? Cocktail shoes: $75; cocktail dress: $175; night out on the town for 2: $250; Vibrant – Radiant Health: PRICELESS! Sure, if you go and buy everything organic & natural in one weekend; then yes it's expensive.   However, I counsel people to slowly (over a period of 3 to 6 months) transition their kitchen pantry into natural & organic. This way they are not out the big expense up front, plus I give them places to buy the best products at lower cost. Who do you want to invest in? You or Washington? What is great skin worth? What about vibrant energy? What is never worrying about taking that blue pill to enhance your libido? To me, all the above are priceless!   As for convenience, what is more convenient?   Going to multiple doctor visits and having multiple ailments then taking pill after pill worrying if you forgot to take one for the day or not? Or taking just a little more effort and knowledge to prepare your food to eliminate doctors? I choose the doctor elimination. If you understand what food can do for you, then you understand how to make it work in your favor.

I want everyone to understand that I am speaking from personal experiences and studies. I am not a doctor of any kind, nor do I claim to treat, diagnose or cure people of any ailment, obesity or disease. So please be advised that this book is intended for educational purposes and to better help you experience a more natural, easy and risk free way to weight loss or weight gain, radiant skin, enhanced libido and better health. I do realize that each person is different and unique and this protocol may not be perfect for everyone. However, the staples I mention here are safe and effective for any person. As with any change of diet, it is recommended that you consult with your natural health care provider before making any decision. This is to ensure your safety and health.

It is my wish that while reading this book you will come to understand the importance of a healthy diet. I also hope you will understand what has happened to our food supply and what is happening now. While reading this book I hope you find benefits in the healthy tips I give you. There are many solutions to your toxic food problem. Solutions are exactly what I offer the world.

I highly recommend that you take the time to research and dig deeper into the subjects I discuss in the following pages.

Remember the only person who really cares about you is YOU. The food industry has no concern if their MSG (mono-sodium glutamate) and GMO (genetically modified organisms) also known as GEF (genetically engineered foods) infested food compromises your health. They have no concern that white sugar and white sodium chloride (they call this 'salt') is poison to the human body or they wouldn't keep making it. Their concern is about padding their pocket books at YOUR expense. This is a huge circle of food to Rx drugs. The more toxic food you eat, the more ailments you will have, hence the numerous drugs you become dependent on. Remember, there is no money in wellness.

I do however, care about the people, I do have concerns and I do want to see people be self-sustaining and eating healthier and saying "Good bye" to the mass market food industry. I care about you and the health of our nation. I want us to be a healthy and thriving nation without relying on the government. This is why I have written this book and 2 more to come. So ask yourself, "What is my health worth to me"?

Psalm 91:9-12; The Lord is my refuge. His angels are with me. Lord give

You see, for we are all our own worst enemy. So be your best friend. Take care of you and your family.

Blessings,

Organic Guru Lynnette Marie

About the Author

Organic Guru Lynnette Marie: Author, Medicine Woman, Minister for the Environment, and YOUR voice for pure food and health freedoms.

As a sought after 'real story' and motivational speaker, Organic Guru Lynnette Marie travels the world sharing healthful information to help you make informed decisions. She graces events such as the Health Freedom Expo: Chicago/ Long Beach, Navel Expo: New York, Heirloom Seed Expo: California & Connecticut, USA Prepares: Missouri, Core Health Conference: Tennessee and in many venues in Mexico. Look for her in an area near you.

Lynnette is the Author of one of the best internationally selling books, 'Fuel for the Body', in which has sold around the world. It was voted the "Best Lay Person" book written on food and health. Fuel for the Body is being distributed by Ingram Content Group, the world's largest and most trusted distributor of physical and digital content. It has been has been endorsed by many health activist, nutritionist and holistic doctors. Lynnette has also published "Lose Weight the Pate Weigh". Look for her other amazing books coming out end of 2015: "What Does Our Creator Have to Say About Our Food & Health" and "Where There Is Life There Is Hope".

Recently, Lynnette commenced her studies and ceremonies to receive her certification to be a Medicine Woman as well as a Minister for the

Environment. A 'Patient Expert', in which she was named by Dr. Ramah Wagner, national speaker and chiropractor. Lynnette studied under the direction of Dr. Ramah Wagner and Dr. Debra Clarke; Acupuncture Therapist of Florida.

After 2 near death experiences with her son, Coty, Lynnette discovered how real food was meant to heal our bodies and cure diseases. Coty suffered 27 surgeries with 7 different surgeons over the course of 15 years. It wasn't until she was connected to a natural practicing doctor in Denver, Co. that she realized diseases CAN be cured. Coty suffered from an "Uncurable" disease: Respiratory Papillomatosis, aka the Human Papilloma Virus (HPV). Lynnette and her husband, Tommy, formed a 501(c)3 Foundation (The Coty Pate Foundation for Respiratory Papillomatosis) on behalf of their son, to help other families suffering, get the appropriate care they needed for their child. A happy note: Coty is alive and thriving at the age of 25, disease and surgery free for over 9 years. He now enjoys his dream of being an international organic chef.

Lynnette suffered from her own kidney surgery at age 8 in which she was on Rx drugs and OTC pills along with yearly emergency room and hospital visits throughout 25 years. It was during her visit and education from her son's doctor in Colorado that she was able to see the difference and the truths of the food and drug industry. From the education she received in Denver, Lynnette buried herself in classes, seminars, lectures and books until she could grasp the way the body was meant to heal itself as well as cleaning toxins out of her environment. Therefore, she set out on a mission to educate and empower the world on the importance of living a toxic free life in order to be disease & ailment free. Lynnette has helped thousands of people around the world lose weight, gain health, reverse diseases and have glowing skin by offering tools for radiant skin, optimum weight & vibrant health.

She is also the Creator & founder of Grass Roots efforts: Fuel for the Body YES T.O.U.R.s (Total Organic Understanding Ride) read more about this amazing mission on her website. As a Minister for the environment, Lynnette, with the help of her staff, founded the Pure Integrity Verified™ Seal of Approval. This is one of the PUREST seals in the WORLD! Find out which companies are truly toxic free!   Organic Guru Lynnette Marie is YOUR pure health activist and takes your voice across the world demanding a toxic free planet! You can finally shop with confidence in knowing you are purchasing from PURE companies. Lynnette and her team say YES! YES to clean food, YES to clean water & YES to clean air!

She is currently involved in communities nation-wide and in Mexico as coordinator of organic festivals, galas and motivational speaker. Lynnette has also been recently named as the Regional Ambassador for the American Anti-Cancer Institute. See more about this amazing center at www.americanaci.org founded by Bob Wright, the author of 'Killing Cancer NOT People'.

Being a PURE health advocate, Lynnette was also selected to be one of the PHresh Super stars / spokes persons for an amazing company: PHresh Products. You will also see Lynnette gracing the website and calendar of Ecco Bella cosmetics and skin care as one of their Brand Ambassadors. She proudly supports companies who have true integrity!

She has been honored with winning the title as 'Ambassador' for America's Outstanding Mom in June of 2012. This honor has entitled Lynnette to reach a completely new audience with her profound message. What better platform than the MOM's pageant to empower women of the WORLD? After all, Moms are the main decision makers for the family when it comes to food and health choices. This is just what she did as Ambassador.

Lynnette enjoys spending valuable time with her family. She has 2 beautiful daughters as well. Jordan Lynnette with 4 beautiful children of her own. So yes, that makes Lynnette a grandmother, but she prefers to be called "Gigi". Her other daughter, Haley Marie is 21 and on her way to College to study physical therapy. Haley and Jordan have brought so much patience to their family while watching their parents tend to their brother's illness. For that, they are deeply appreciated. Lynnette and her husband, Tommy, enjoyed being Foster Parents for abused and neglected children for a few years. This was only due to the inspiration of their 3 loving children wanting to bring helpless children into their home to take care of them. They went through non-state funded organizations such as Agape of Memphis, TN.

She is also a huge activist for spreading God's message to the world. By following the word of God, one has the tools they need to live a life of longevity, purity and integrity.

"The better you take care of your body, the better your body takes care of YOU". Lynnette Marie

LIVE HAPPY. BE PURE!

> *"A healthy nation can conquer all, but a sick nation will surely fall"*
> *Lynnette Marie*

Lynnette's mission is to inspire, enlighten and empower the world to arm themselves with great nutrition. She truly cares for your health.

Inspirations

My inspirations come from my willingness to understand how our bodies were meant to heal themselves naturally.

I have been inspired by my friend and re-known Dr. Ramah Wagner of Wagner Chiropractic Center in central Florida. She is the author of the 'Health of Business' – a must read for anyone wanting a healthy revolution! Ramah has inspired me to be who I am, to just go and finish my books and to not be fearful or intimidated by doctors, scientist or people I think are superior. She has taught me to understand myself. Ramah has shared the stage with many well- known doctors as well as Suzanne Sommers.

Also I have been inspired by my friend, Dr. Debra Clarke of the White Peacock Interactive Center. Debra is an Acupuncture Physician of Central Florida. She has inspired me to spread my wings and "teach" people from my experiences. She tells me we all learn from each other and my experience with the "real" foods and real world brings better understanding to her clinic. I have studied and taken direction and training from my good friend, Debra Clarke as well as worked with Dr. Ramah in their clinics.

My children Coty, Jordan & Haley have also inspired me to make a better world, a better healthier world for their future and their children's future. They are the reason I try to better myself and empower humanity. We have had our medical experiences in the western medicine and MSG, GMO and GEF infested world.

I have come to realize that American's are so conditioned in to eating the "Big Pharma" foods and taking their meds.   Therefore, I ventured out to seek answers. Answers are exactly what I got. These answers led me to study more into the food world. By using food to work for our bodies, we have a much higher chance of fighting off diseases, obesity and many ailments and even curing the diseases.

When we look all around us and we see half or more of the nation on OTC drugs, Rx drugs and seeing psychiatrist, we have to wonder what in the world is going on. We see obesity at an absurd number and we see more and more vaccinations and so many diseased, sick and nearly dead people. Autism is at an outrageous explosion as well as the dreaded cancer. Is it any wonder we can even function as a human society? If you want to know what the culprit is to all our ailments, then study this enlightening book. You will have an entire new outlook on how food was intended to be. It's NOT rocket science! There are many problems we face in our world. I like to provide solutions for those problems.

"The problem is not the problem, the problem is your attitude about the problem". Captain Jack Sparrow.

We can overcome any problem.   Ha, yes, I know, but you've just gotta love Captain Jack's analogies! Much love to you all.

Thank You

There are so many people to thank. But first and foremost, I am most thankful to my Creator in Heaven for giving me the knowledge and steadfastness to be able to present these series of books to the public.

I then want to thank my dear best friend Tommy Pate, for understanding my desire. Also for giving me the support to be able to open our organic retail shop. This enabled me to pursue my passion for educating the world on organic and sustainable living. He is the reason the T.O.U.R.s keep pedaling on and my events keep manifesting.

Next, I want to give a huge thank you to my children, Coty, Jordan & Haley for understanding me a little better after they have grown into amazing adults.

Also, if it weren't for my dad, Harold Hagar passing down his genes of the ability to keep pressing on when times were down, I would not be in this position today with information to pass on to you. My dad gave me hope and the fun side of life. He encouraged me to always have a smile on my face no matter what. I love you Dad!

Lastly, thank you to all my fans & friends I have acquired since the printing of my first edition book. Thank you to all of the organizations who have invited me to speak at their festivals and conferences.

Thank you for your continued questions and support you have shown over the past few years. I truly each and every one of you.

Lynnette

Introduction

I have written this short book to get you on your way to a healthier, happier you. Fuel for the Body is an easy to follow instruction guide plus the SECRET essential staples to give you a jump start to eating more nutritious to have vibrant health, radiant skin and that ultimate sexual enhancement. Losing weight is just an added 'side effect' benefit you will enjoy if you need to lose. However, if you need to gain weight, this will be accomplished as well. If you are tired of counting calories, fat grams and points and you are tired of diets that just do not work, then this book is for you.

I don't even like to call this a "weight loss" book as it's so much more than that. It is a total nutrition book with the "side effect" of pure blissful health! So how would you like that for a side effect? It's also a guide for beautiful radiant skin, energized health and awesome sex! By FUELING your body with proper nutrition, all of these things can be obtained. Yes, if you are seeking that secret to enhanced libido, THIS is your answer!

I do not buy into the obesity is a disease mentality. I do, however believe you ARE what you eat. I used to believe that overweight people just ate themselves that way or they just couldn't say no. I believed that because I, myself, would always have to be careful of what I ate as I have the genes to become very overweight and have easily put on several extra pounds. I have come to understand after studying and researching the food industry for the past few years, that it is possible for people to be overweight by no "real" fault of their own. It is possible for people to be sluggish all the time. It is possible to lose your sex drive. It is possible to have progressively aging skin. All this by no real fault of the individual. Why? Well, because of the wonders of the food industry. The food industry and big pharma has led us to believe that all the processed foods are actually good for us. The fact of the matter is, they have tainted and adulterated the food to leave no nutritional value what so ever. The MSG, GMO and GEF foods simply trigger our brain into being hungry and have crazy sugar cravings. Remember, if you are drinking a diet soda and having a candy bar or snack cake, that's not going to cut it! So read on to find out what all of this means.

'Fuel for the Body' is written to help you get acquainted with eating more nutritiously. You will find that after following this protocol, you will want more information on other foods to add to your daily diet. You will have more energy without the after crash. You will have better metabolism. Some are experiencing lower cholesterol and lower blood sugar levels and of course lowering their blood pressure. Others do indeed gain that awesome libido they seem to lose at certain times in their lives. Then others are experiencing the fabulous skin they always dreamed of! This is more than just weight loss or weight gain, it is a way of life.

Most Americans do not understand the way food can work for them and not against them. We will cover that subject in the following book. Most Americans have a hard time breaking out of the rut they have been in for so many years due to lack of education about the food they already consume. By doing exactly what I tell you to do in this book, you will experience less and less cravings of the bad sugars, starches and fats. You then will be excited and want to be more educated about how other foods will benefit you.

These unique staples I mention to you have been tried and tested by myself, clients and friends. Therefore, no animals were ever tested using my 'experiments', ha! I came up with this regimen several years ago after trying to help a couple of my friends to lose weight and overcome some health issues. After trying various foods, one at a time, and none were doing quite like I wanted, I stumbled across one very important staple. I first tried it myself and was very pleased with the taste and the energy it gave me and the controlled appetite I felt. I then gave it to my friends to try. They experienced the same as I. So I began my quest to find even more healthy foods to add to their diets. I was on a quest to not only find weight loss foods, but to get good health benefits as well. After studying the wonderful health benefits of the 1st staple, I was astonished at what I found. I wanted to compliment this food with other fat burning foods. I did my due research and added 2 more staples to my diet as well as my friends' diets. The other staples proved to attack the bad fats and help the digestion track which is vital for any healthy diet.

The mentioned staples are something every household should NEVER be without. I use these every day of my life. I do it for healthy maintenance. I just use a lesser amount than what I recommend clients who need to lose weight. These staples are so essential, that children can consume them. In fact, I have recommended to parents who cannot get their child to eat, to give a small amount of 2 of the staples.

I now invite you to start enjoying the healthy alternative to eating faux food. You really are what you eat!

I am sure you will be delighted with the content of Fuel for the Body. If you would like further consultation on how to completely change the way you view food, I am available for phone or skype consults as well as in person. Please feel free to call to book an appointment with one of my assistants. You may also feel free to call with any questions you may have. Keeping in mind, I am a Patient Expert, Certified Medicine Woman, mentor and healthy nutrition Consultant/Coach. I am not a doctor, nurse or scientist. I do not give medical advice. I do advise you however, to consult with your natural health care practitioner before changing any part of your daily diet. I do recommend you getting your blood sugar and cholesterol checked during your eating changes.

Fuel for the Body is a "jump start" for you to be on your way to goal achievement. My following books will give you more insight of other foods to incorporate into your diet. You will become more and more familiar with what you are eating and how they affect your body.

Here's to your good health and eating habits!

You are now on your way to a happier healthier, radiant and sexier YOU with, Fuel for the Body!

LIVE HAPPY. BE PURE!

Testimonials

When I started Lynnette's program, my blood pressure was 150/100 and I had 50 pounds to lose. I felt miserable and was tired all the time. I just had my recheck with the doctor and the results speak for themselves. My blood pressure was 136/84 and I had lost 8 pounds. Everyone has commented that I have more pep and seem to glow. Lynnette REALLY knows her stuff. I was holding water and she told me to try Celtic Sea Salt. I lost 4 pounds in one week!! I know it was the salt water. Thanks Lynnette!

Shari Chuchla; FL 2010

I was around 196 I am now 180. I have more energy where before if I exerted any during the day I would be wiped out for a few days. I haven't got sick so far this winter which is very unusual for me, I was usually sick all the time. The more in shape I get the more energized I feel. I know I'm going to get to my goal! I just went to my lung doctor, he said my influx capacity went from 76 percent to 87 much better from last year. He told me to keep up the good work. My size right now is 14 on the smaller side of 14 if there is such a thing. Top size is large. This past year I started using organic and naturals in my business. I've struggled with my weight most all my life. I've struggled with a disease that left me fatigued and sick for the past seven years. I'm so great-full for this opportunity of being chosen for this challenge of getting healthy. I feel better now than I have in years. I believe this is just the beginning of a lifelong way of life now. Thank you so much Lynette, I think you have touched a lot of lives with your book and your shining enthusiasm. May God Bless you and be with you.

Denise Butcher; FL 2010

On January 3, 2010, I weighed in @ 327lbs. and wore a size tight 26. Since beginning Lynnette Pate's protocol in the Pate Weigh, I have had awesome results! My current pant size is now a 24!

Yay, and I am still dropping pounds. My energy level is astounding! I no longer come home from school exhausted and lay in bed. I actually work, either in the garden or at home until bed time!
Thank you, Lynnette, for the journey thus far!
Shawn Dingman; FL 2010

My weight before starting the Pate Weigh was 239, and I am currently at 189 and still shrinking! My big issues were headaches and monthly issues. My headaches have been almost non-existent. Some unexpected but pleasant side effects have been that my skin has dramatically cleared up. I think that is why people keep telling me that I look like I'm glowing! Also, I have so much energy that I have a hard time getting rid of it at times. Thank you, Lynnette, for enlightening me on the truth about foods!

Gidget Blunt; FL 2010

"Lynnette, I wanted to thank you for being so caring and compassionate and one of the first person that God used to inspire me in my new path as a Holistic Health Coach! Your book Fuel For The Body is really powerful and eye opening and I felt like you were talking to me, I enjoyed it very much! Your passion is so contagious and love for the truth is sowing a lot seeds in the minds and hearts of people. God bless you in your calling and give you the wisdom and grace to keep going. Blessings"!

-Talia Alanis, VA

"Best two things I ever learned from OrganicGuru Lynnette Pate- 1. use lots of virgin coconut oil 2. Get rid of diet sodas forever. I think people are catching on to the MYTH of diet sodas, Lynnette. This guy just plain says THEY KILL YOU".

-Tammy Caldwell de Leeuw; CA

My friend Devoni let me use her book, Fuel for the Body! This book has helped to change my life! Thanks Lynnette"!

-Laura Headrick; LA

About 2 years ago I made the decision to really start paying attention to what I was eating, looking for weight loss and overall better health. At least a year ago I came across the Organic Guru Lynnette Pate and her bicycle tour for organic freedom across America with her book Fuel for the Body. I was hooked, one because the book was very easy to read and refer back to laying out simple things anyone could do to maintain better health and two because she was confirming everything I knew and felt in my heart about our food supply. The very simple changes that I have made in my daily routine help me maintain my blood sugar, blood pressure and weight. I still have a way to go but making simple adjustments in my daily routine has taken me miles from where I used to be! I feel so much better and knowing that I am taking my health in my own hands is a big motivator. Lynnette is a warrior for clean food and I cannot wait to see the progress we are all sure to make in our food health!

~Heather Collette; MS

"I have been friends with Ms. Pate for about 3 years now. And she eloquently and clearly points out all of the reasons why some in the American public are suffering from an assortment of ailments. She points out that good sound nutrition is a MUST for building a better body, along with exercise and proper supplementation. She also reminds us that most Americans have no idea what they're putting into their bodies, and the toxic and lethal chemicals that they are ingesting into their bodies. The long-term ramifications of doing just that is enormous that results in numerous maladies ranging from chronic illnesses, cancer, heart disease, diabetes, stroke, etc. I would HIGHLY recommend reading her book because not only is it very easy to read and understand, but also, fills the reader in on exactly how to acquire proper nutritional habits and lifestyle changes that will result in a higher quality of life."

Shahid Mufti; MI

"Lynette, just wanted to let you that this protocol IS DA BEST. 1/20/2010 will be week 3 and I feel awesome. I have lost 4lbs since the protocol and losing more. With the exercise techniques that Kris from Omni Fitness of Fruitland Park Leesburg, has showed are easy too. Taking the items of protocol have become 2nd nature. If I don't take them I don't feel right. Thanks so much to all who have contributed to this protocol. Without this I don't know if I was going to ever fit in my wedding dress!   Whom ever is looking to lose weight safely & organic style I say: *LOSE WEIGHT THE PATE WEIGH*"

Edwich Green: Florida

"Started your new class on April 1.   Unbelievable   first   nite. Learned tons and am applying it all. Expect to enjoy highr energy, less hunger and nutrition impact at the cellular level, In short, I expect to feel better and look better fairly quickly. Thanks for sharing your hard-fought wisdom and experience.

Anyone missing your classes is a shame. Incredible information for the price of a decent meal out.

David Williams: Florida

Lynnette - thank you so much for sharing your knowledge - I'm learning something new every day! I have more energy and I'm not hungry all the time - WHO KNEW - well, apparently you did - and thank you! I look forward to the journey of becoming healthier!
I know we're all going to gain a better understanding of how to be healthy and wise in 2010!

Lynn Anderson: Florida

Fuel for the Body

Your tools to optimum weight,
radiant skin and vibrant health.
Enhanced libido as well!

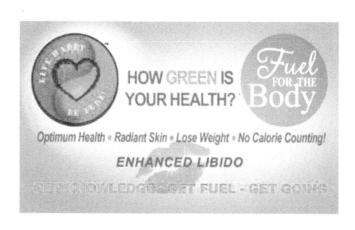

Fuel for the Body

Simple, natural additions to a more healthier, energetic, radiant and happier YOU!

This is for everyone. Even if you don't need to lose weight, this is for all aspects of health. The ultimate body guide!

Are you tired of counting calories, fat grams, carbohydrates or points??? Well stop counting these vital nutrients! Let's worry about how many toxins are lurking in your body from consuming unnatural foods. What if I told you that you can eat what you want and never deprive yourself of amazing foods you love? What if I told you that you can do this and still have the weight of your dreams, the energy you long for, the skin you desire and the most amazing health ever? You don't have to worry about being sick, tired, over-weight or on Rx drugs, if you eat the right foods and take my advice seriously. Are you sick of being sick and tired of being tired? Have you lost your libido? Is your skin the one you love to live in? It is up to you to write the story of the way your life will end or begin. You can choose to grow diseases or you can choose to prevent diseases. You can choose to use these tools of healthful information to arm yourself with or you can choose to keep doing what you are doing and keep getting the results you are getting. I will be planting the seed for you. It will be up to you to nourish your seed.

This is NOT a diet, fad or quick fix to your weight or health problems. Nor is this book only about losing weight. This is a short memo to help you get on your way to vibrant more radiant health. I will discuss more life enhancing facts in my following book. There are NO magic wands or "miracle" pills to remedy your health and weight problems. This is simply a way of life. You are just adding life-enhancing natural and organic staples to feed your body of what it has been deprived of. You will have "Fuel for the Body". Diets, pills or any quick fix way to lose weight will only harm you in the long run. Sure you can lose weight fast, but will you be healthy? Will you keep it off? What are the long term effects? The only sure fire way to lose weight and KEEP it off is living a HEALTHY lifestyle. This means you must exercise, eat your organic foods and drink your purified water and juices. This is a life style not a fad diet or a corner cutting technique. Do not take short cuts. It's just not worth it! Why not lose weight or gain weight, be healthy, have glowing skin, a happier sex life and live longer? You can do just that, simple and easy. No 'pre-made meals' to buy and no blue print systems. Nor will I impose on you some marketing system of supplements you have to "buy" in to and be billed month after month.

I did not want to make this complicated at all, nor did I want to mislead you into taking some pill or supplement that may or may not work. I have tested these foods and routine on my own self, friends and clients...so needless to say, absolutely NO animals were ever our guinea pigs. Only tested on real

HUMANS! After trial and error and studying different foods and knowing what certain foods do for the body, I have come up with a "jump start" plan to get you on the right track of eating a more nutritious way. After you have incorporated these essential staples into your diet, you will start discovering how less hungry you are, how much more energy you have and how much less you will crave those "fake" foods. We like to call these "fake" foods - GMO, (genetically modified organisms) MSG, (mono sodium glutamate) pesticide and preservative infested items that the FDA likes to call food! Remember to always keep in mind this is not a 'one size fits all' method. However, it has not failed with the clients whom have incorporated this lifestyle over the past few years. You must know what health issues you have, how you became unhealthy and how to work to eliminate certain foods until you can become entirely toxic free.

Taking diet pills, laxatives and starving yourself will give you unwelcoming side effects such as; constipation, constant gas pains, anemia, risk of heart attack and many other ailments. Who wants to deal with or has time for costly side effects? Then you have to take another pill to remedy that ailment. UGH! Certainly not me! The only "side effects" you are going to experience by adding these staples to your daily diet will be...WEIGHT LOSS, (if needed or weight gain for that matter) enhanced LIBIDO, GLOWING SKIN and IMPROVED HEALTH! You will then be so excited of your stamina and success that you will not want to put any of that 'faux' food into your body anymore. While I did not want to overload your mind with too many lifestyle changes, I know that after incorporating these foods, you will want more information on how to actually be ALIVE and be HEALTHY instead of just living. What would you do to not have to worry about what you eat? Not have to worry about calories or fat grams or being allergic? When you transition to a toxic free life style, your worries will be over. You can have that chocolate and eat it too!

Why Be Toxin Free?

Your health is your wealth! I know how important real food and exercise is to the body. I know because, although I have never been severely overweight, I have had my battles with keeping my weight at one size. I used to be religious in going to the gym and working out at home with weights and gym sets. I got my body in great 'looking' shape. Wow, I thought I had it figured out. I looked amazing and my clothes fit perfectly. However, something was not right. I seemed to look great on the outside, but I did not feel well on the inside. Hmmm, how could this be? I was bloated with gas pains, indigestion and constipation. Wonder why? Well gee, I was not properly nourishing my insides! Sure, I was eating "healthy" with no sweets and low calories, low carbs and so on. I just didn't have the missing link then. I was still filling my body full of environmental toxins and polluted food from the food industry. It wasn't till years later when I turned my house upside down to change to all organic food that the 'ah ha' light bulb went off. I have tried it all: fad diets, pills and no fat diets only to find disappointment and frustration with constipation, bloating and poor circulation. I have tried all the tricks out there. Believe me, NONE of them work! I did have rapid weight loss with one pill I took. However, my health paid for it and I put on more weight than I started with after I quit taking them. I am prone to be overweight, as it runs on my mother's side of the family. I have always had to watch what I eat, that is until now. Now that I have completely changed the way I think and the way I view food.

I understand that God put food on this planet for our nourishment and health. God gave us food to work for us NOT us work for food. Our Creator knew what we needed to survive. However, the food industry and 'big pharma' have been slowly taking away our God given survival foods. We do not make food like we used to! Back to the basics with natural, non-polluted, God given foods is what I am talking about here. Organic and toxic free are the KEY words. Organic is not a 'new age' yuppy kind of life style. Organic simply means going back to the basic non-chemical, non-genetically modified organisms and non-hormone growth injections. Organic means, real pure food! That's it. You can taste the difference in eating organic foods. These foods have far more nutrition than man altered foods. Eating organic provides you with the living bacteria and enzymes to satisfy your body. You get all the nutrients you need by eating organic and natural which will eliminate the need for sugary cravings and excessively over indulging. You will soon realize that eating organic foods will lift your spirits and raise your energy levels as well as prevent some ailments you may complain about now.

I know some of you reading this are saying, "Yeah right Lynnette, organic is just a new craze out here and I have been eating non-organic all my life and

I'm just fine". No, organic has been around since the beginning of time. Only then, there was no need to call it organic since the toxic pesticides and herbicides did not exist then. It was just called FOOD. Food was grown in the purest and natural state. As far as you eating non-organic foods all your life, you tell me, are you currently struggling with weight, sickness, fatigue, disease or any ailment? Are you taking or have you been prescribed prescriptions drugs or taking over the counter drugs? It is very possible and very achievable to live free from Rx drugs or OTC drugs. It is possible to live an entire sick free and ailment free life. Remember this, 3 percent of the population are very lucky they were born with astounding genes. This 3% can go their entire lives eating junk foods, non-organic food and doing whatever the heck they want without ever having any health or weight issues what so ever. So that leaves the rest of the 97 percent of the population. What about these people? They have ailments, sickness, weight issues and so on. Unless you are one of the 3% few, then you should consider what you are really eating!

I understand that everyone is different and unique. Therefore, you have to know your own body and understand how food nourishes different ailments. I also do not buy into the idea that obesity is a "disease" that you need medication for. I used to believe that people have the power to control their eating habits and needed to pull away from the table. I still believe that, to an extent. I believe that one should know better than to have a "diet" drink while eating a twinkie or candy bar! Speaking of diet drinks, get those OUT of your life! Diet drinks are the worst culprit in obesity, high blood sugar and cholesterol.

I do feel that our government has conditioned the majority of Americans into eating what "they" consider to be healthy. Therefore, I now believe that not every person who is over weight is completely at fault of their own. They are eating what the government deems "healthy" for us. They have been deprived of true facts about foods and toxins. I mean look at our nation, we are the most over fed and under nourished country in the world. Good grief, with all the abundance of food we have here an America and all the top doctors of the world and our wonderful world of technology, why are we such a sick nation? Yes, I love our country, but you have got to understand, we have a serious problem on our hands. Remember the old saying, "If you keep doing what you are doing, then you will keep getting what you are getting"? Well the same goes for food. We will discuss false teachings in my 3rd book, 'Stop Eating the Blue Pill'. But don't let this hinder you, as I believe always, where there is life there is hope! Therefore, educating yourself about real foods and toxins lurking in the food industry foods, you can better arm yourself with nutritional information to help you to make informed decisions.

You are what you eat, meaning, that if you continually put chemicals, preservatives and pesticides in your body you will reap the seeds that you have sown. Our bodies were not meant to consume these foreign ingredients. Our kidneys and liver can only filter so much during our life time. I will leave the functions of body organs to trusted healthcare providers to explain to you. We cannot properly digest these chemicals, so our bodies reject them sending our intestines into overload. This wreaks havoc on our digestive system creating fatty deposits being stored and clogged in our body. Our intestines then cannot properly expel our waste. It is very important to have waste elimination 2 to 4 times per day. However, the Standard American Diet (SAD) has confined Americans to only 1 bowel movement per day and sometimes even 1 every other day. This is certainly not healthy. This causes excess fat build up and tons of horrific toxins in the colon and possibly getting in the blood stream. This is a factor in weight gain. It also causes fatigue and other sickness and diseases. A clean colon is a happy colon. Speaking of which, did you know that the average person carries in their colon 8 lbs. of toxic waste per year? Yes, this is true! "Wow, you mean to tell me I have 8 lbs. of sludge inside me"? Yes indeed. Just imagine carrying 8 lbs. of sludge inside you year after year. Think of all the pounds you are adding up for several years at 8 lbs. per year! Wow, it's no wonder we are sick and overweight. Of course some of this toxic waste is eliminated throughout the year, but most of it sticks with you. You can rid yourself of unwanted pounds rather quickly by simply doing a body or colon cleanse with natural nutrients. Although, I do recommend getting a colonics once per year.

Especially if you have never had one and you are just now coming from the toxic infested food world. These are very natural enhancers to safely help you eliminate that horrible toxic sludge in your colon. Look for a trusted day spa in your area and you will be sure to find the information you need.

I say all this to let you know that I understand your concerns such as: "I've tried to lose weight steadily and just can't get it off" or "I only eat small portions and I exercise a few times per week and nothing works". You can do all these things, but if you are not eating the proper way or the proper foods, then you are wasting your time. The chemicals we ingest harm our metabolism and thyroid, especially our thyroid. When these two things are out of whack, then your whole body malfunctions. This is why it is so important to nourish your body with God given foods that were meant for human consumption. With these simple staples you will be introduced to, you will find much of your digestion problems and ailments remedied.

Want a long healthy life so you can see your grand kids grow up? What price can you put on your health? Living a healthy life style will afford you a quality of life that surpasses any material wants. The importance of living an organic life style is extremely important to our children and our children's future. Remember, we are borrowing the planet from our children. As of right now, this is the only planet we have to survive on. Your body is the only place you have to live in. Therefore, taking care of these two temples is of the utmost importance. So think on these things. Invest in YOU. Let your food be your insurance policy and your health care reform.

Let's Talk About Exercise A Bit

Remember, it is very important to incorporate exercise into your daily routine. Exercising will compliment the healthy foods you eat, just as healthy foods will compliment exercise. It's all about balance. You can't have one without the other. Exercising can be fun, in fact it should be fun. There are so many things you can do during each day to keep your body active. You can do simple 15 minute stretches in the morning before jetting off to work or doing household chores. Taking the stairs instead of the elevator is great exercise. We Americans under estimate the power of walking. Our bodies were created to walk and they were created to walk long distances. So walk, walk, walk your way to a life of healthiness. Looking for that wonderful closest parking space near the grocery or department store? No need to waste precious exercising time, just park farther away and WALK. Walking will do the body good! Enroll in Yoga or Pilates. These 2 exercises are perfect for flexibility, posture and healthy breathing. They also help maintain the body's ability to control the appetite and keep the muscles strengthened. Yes, good for both men & women. We will discuss the importance of these 2 exercises in future books. You might also want to check out a rebounder, this is a mini trampoline. Rebounders are great for strengthening the ankles and preventing fluid build-up on the legs. They are great for the lymph nodes as well to keep them flushed. Rebounding is also good for keeping you regular. You can use your rebounder 1 to several times a day. Rebounding is easily done by watching your TV program or talking on the phone to clients or friends. Do your research on good quality rebounders such as the cellerciser. The benefits of exercising on a mini trampoline are astonishing and have been promoted significantly within the last decade. It is a unique exercise in which a weightless state is achieved at the top of each jump and landing achieves twice the force of gravity on each bounce. This shift in gravity benefits every muscle and cell of the body and provides huge benefits to the lymph system.

On studying the benefits of rebounding, NASA found that a 150-pound individual spending one-hour on a rebounder will burn more calories than the same person jogging for an hour!

So you see, you don't have to spend a fortune on gyms or clubs just to get your daily exercise. Of course, going to any gym will give you more motivation. I do recommend light weight training for added metabolism and fat burning ability. You can purchase free-weights at local sporting good stores. If you already have a gym membership, great, use it! Or check out books such as '*Home Workout Bible' by Brad Shoenfeld* and my friend and personal trainer: Donovan Green, author of: 'No Excuse Fitness'. Donovan is also the personal trainer to Dr. Oz! His motto is: "*My mission is to* eliminate your EXCUSES to not live a healthy life style and increase your awareness of the importance

of living a healthier lifestyle. By the time I'm done with you there will be no more EXCUSES"! "Stop making excuses and LIVE"! Let's take a peak at what Donovan has to offer you.

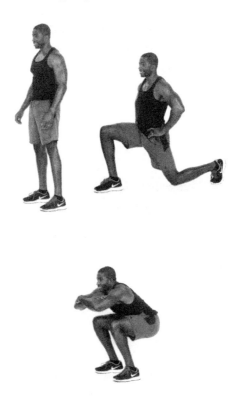

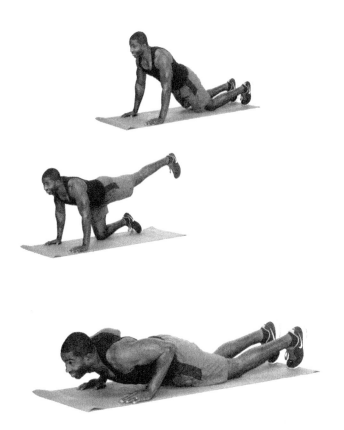

Each exercise must be repeated for a total of 30 seconds. Do as many rounds as possible within 20 minutes

Squats

Stand with your feet a little bit more than shoulder width apart. Push your butt back and pretend you were sitting back into a seat. Cross your hands in front of your chest and bend your knees bringing your butt parallel to the floor and knees bent at 90 degrees. Exhale as you press your heels through the ground bringing your body back to standing position

*Note: make sure to keep your knees behind your toes.

Reverse lunges

Stand with your feet shoulder width apart and your hand placed on your hips. Keep your back straight and lift your chest as if you were proud. Step back with your left leg as you bend your knees at 90 degrees. Exhale as you return back to standing position and repeat on the right side.

*Note: Do not let your knees hit the floor.

Modified push ups

Start with your knees on the floor. Press your palms into the ground using your arms to support your body weight. Bend your elbows to lower your body to the floor keeping your stomach muscles tight. Exhale and push your body back away from the floor.

Jack Knife

Lay with your feet separated and arm placed out on the sides of your body. Take a deep breath in and then exhale as you lift your body up to the shape of the letter V. lower your body back down to the ground and repeat.

*Note: make sure to keep your stomach muscles tight and avoid tension on your lower back.

Butt lifts

Assume position on all fours. Press the weight into your palms and shift some of weight to your left knee. Extend your right leg out behind you tightening your gluteus. Lift your leg up and down. You should feel a burning sensation in your right gluteus. You can benefit a great deal more from Donovan's website: www.projectslimdown.com *"Your body is just a body, until you make it a temple".* *Donovan Green*

For those of you who have desk jobs, you can still exercise during the day. As you sit at your desk typing or making phone calls, be aware of your posture. Posture makes a difference in your breathing, fatigue and aches. When you have good posture, you can breathe better therefore allowing your body to better detoxify. Speaking of deep breathing, oxygen therapy at oxygen bar centers is a great way to deeply inhale purified oxygen. Good purified oxygen allows our bodies to detoxify naturally releasing bad toxin build up. This allows our body's cells to work in harmony. You should also take note that free radicals, bacteria and cancer cells cannot survive in a well oxygenated environment. Also practice deep breathing exercises and meditation. These are great ways to get great oxygen to your lungs. Have an office job? While sitting at your desk, if you are typing, suck in your stomach as if you were trying to touch your back with it and hold for a few seconds then release. Repeat this several times during the day. You will start to make this a habit that you can't break. It will become 2nd nature and will be actually fun! This is a perfect way to flex your abdomen muscles and strengthen them. You can also do this simple exercise in your car on your way to work or play.

Exercise is an important daily activity whether you are walking, rebounding, dancing, yoga or hard work labor. Any and all exercise is beneficial for a healthy lifestyle and healthy body. Typically it is best, if you are working out and getting your daily exercise, if you do it first thing in the morning on an empty stomach. First of all, this enables you to "get it out of the way" and it does not run into your daily agenda or hinder your exercise due to lack of time. Secondly, it enables your body to power more efficiently with the metabolism working harder to burn fat better. Then you can simply 'fuel' your body with a delightful nutritious breakfast such as boiled, scrambled or omelet eggs, smoothie, hot Yerba Mate, blue berries and or salmon. Anyway, you get the gist of a nutritious breakfast, or at least you will by the time you complete this book. However, feel free to get your daily exercise at any time of the day.

Meditation is a great way to relieve stress, and stress is a huge factor in disease and obesity. So meditate in yoga settings, in your own peaceful retreat tucked in your home or out on you lake on a dock or where ever you can have complete solace and quiet. Then follow with yoga, stretches or palates. Purifying the body, mind and spirit is essential to a vibrant life style. Meditation is great to help you really focus on your ability to understand what you are eating. This helps you to get your days off to a more energized start as well. Try making your own Zen Garden in your back yard. These are very easy to do and helps focus on concentration. Check out the web for back yard zen gardens. Plus practicing yoga and meditation will help your mind relax. Meditation is great for suppressing blood pressure, boosting immunity, balances intuition, decreases headaches, increases happiness, helps to focus, raises energy and helps to become more creative. We simply must slow down our life style. We must stop and just breathe a while.

YOU are beautiful and you can make a difference. You are loved and you can send love. You have the ability to do and accomplish anything you desire. You can live a life of healthiness, happiness and radiance". L. Marie

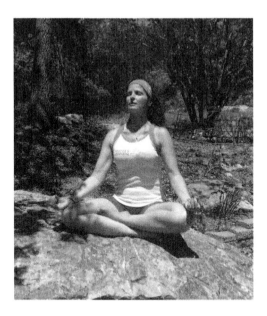

Just remember to get your daily exercise! For bodily exercise brings the divine increase of physical strength. No need to run yourself to death or jog all the time. Horse riding, gardening, bicycling and sports are great. Just do something EVERYDAY! Check out your local bike teams, a lot of them welcome new comers and do it for recreation as well as competitive. This will give you like minds and they are so encouraging and uplifting. Remember to always: LIVE HAPPY. BE PURE

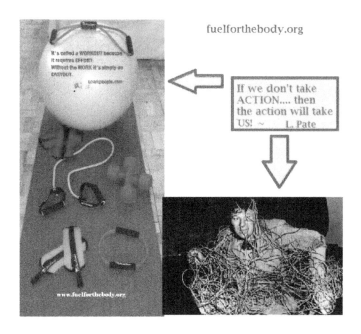

fuelforthebody.org

If we don't take ACTION.... then the action will take US! ~   L. Pate

Who Is Your Role Model?

I do practice what I preach. Or you could say, I preach what I practice. I use the products I mention religiously. I just use a smaller portion than I recommend for someone needing to lose weight. I use the items I mention for skincare and for exercise.

Have you ever looked at people whom are giving you advice yet they don't appear to be following it themselves? Do you wonder why you should take their advice of putting on make-up when they look like a clown themselves? Do you wonder if that skincare she is trying to sell you really works when her skin looks like dot to dot games? Lastly, do you wonder why that 'weight loss' plan your consultant is telling you to do does NOT work on him/her because they are twice or 5 times your size or totally look out of shape? Good grief! There are so many people out there with the "cure for all" or they have all the answers for everyone. All these people look the way they do because:

a) They are NOT using a good product or routine
b) They do NOT practice what they preach
c) They just simply do NOT know what they are talking about.

I am here to tell you, no – I am here to show you
what works. Why and how? Because I PRACTICE
what I preach. No, I am not the best thing out here
or have the perfect situation for everyone, but I am
not overweight, out of shape or have unhealthy
looking skin. You could say it's just 'my genes'.
Some of that could play a part in my appearance.
However, I work very hard (actually it is very easy
and a way of life for me now) to stay in the shape I
am in and have clear, glowing skin. I could easily be
overweight, unhealthy and poor skin. I choose NOT
to, I choose to take care of my body so my body will
take care of me. It is simply a way of life. You have
to rid your mind of the way it has been taught on
TV, radio or department and grocery stores. You
have to realize what makes common sense. So why
not take advice from someone who actually looks
the part?! I say all of this for humor and because it
is the truth. I have ran into so many people who are
skin care "experts", weight loss "consultants" and so
on. I just look at them and wonder what planet they
are from? You know the ones I am talking about. I
have seriously met some 'health coaches' ,
'nutritionist' and others who looked like they had
been sucked dry of any moisture their body ever had
and look so wrinkled, but they wanted to show how
to reverse the signs of aging. Also they were
smokers while they were supposedly 'health
coaches'. Keep in mind, I do know there are some
great health coaches out there who are very over
weight and look very unhealthy, however they
themselves have just now entered this organic world
and they are on their road to complete healthiness

and are losing weight or gaining health as they teach others. So I am not only at first sight judging someone, I get to know them and then make my mind up. However, I do believe in appearances.

Seriously, if you take my advice and sincerely evaluate your eating habits you are going to see results for the better. You will want to learn more ways to eat healthy. Mainly, you will feel better and will feel better about what you feed your family. You will also be able to make informed decisions.

I am NOT a doctor, nurse or scientist or anything of the sort. I am a simple, ordinary, normal person who wants a better way of life. I am not telling you this is a diet, nor am I telling you that this is the perfect answer for your weight problems or health concerns. So obviously none of these statements or protocols have been approved or regulated by the FDA. Frankly, I would rather the FDA stay out of my food. Speaking of the FDA, have you ever wondered why food and drugs are in the same administration? I will address this question in my following book as well.

Speaking of which, the staples and advice I mention in this book are absolutely my own advice, my own experience and my own way of life. This is what I and my family believe, this is what we live. These are foods that have great benefits other than weight loss. These are foods that nourish and 'fuel' the body and are healthy for a child to consume. We will cover the other health benefits on the pages following.

Therefore, I ask you again, what role model would you prefer to follow? Someone who is fat, sick and nearly dead and has funky looking skin?   Or someone who inspires you and tries to continue learning from others? I do believe we can all teach each other. So take it from me, someone who has been on the 'other side' of the fence in the toxic infested world. My results speak for themselves. Be sure and study my skin care chapter in here for some great tips on really radiant skin and ways to reverse the signs of aging.

Drinking Matters

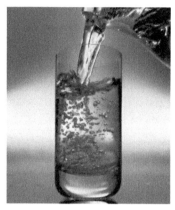

Compliments of royalty free pictures

It is very important to keep yourself well hydrated during the day. Over 70% of our body is water, and we need clean water every day to rejuvenate our system and flush out toxins. Water is the foundation of our health. However, I do not believe in over indulging in liquid drinks all day. I do not even follow the rule of eight to 10 8oz. glasses of water per day. (unless I have a lot of toxic build up straining my kidneys) I drink my 3 to 5 cups of hot herbal and green teas and some good purified yet mineralized water in between. I personally use the Nikken and the Berkey water filtering systems. I do encourage you to drink your daily glasses of clean and mineralized water each day as this keeps the blood flowing and the toxins more easily eliminated.

Squeeze a lemon or a lime in the water to enhance the flavor. Plus this is a great way to cleanse the cells. Also, I do recommend drinking Yerba Mate tea every day or some type of green or white or herbal teas every day. I have a wide variety of herbal and green teas, from yerba mate, to fresh herbs to yogi teas. Yerba mate was discovered centuries ago by the indigenous people in South America and has been revered as the "drink of the gods" and consumed to enhance, vitality, clarity, and well-being. With 24 vitamins and minerals, 15 amino acids, 11 polyphenols, caffeine, and is high in antioxidants, yerba mate triumphs as nature's most balanced stimulant.

Of the six commonly used stimulants in the world--yerba mate, coffee, tea, kola nut, cocoa, and guarana--yerba mate is the healthiest, delivering both energy and nutrition. It helps stimulate focus and clarity*, boosts physical energy*, traditionally used to support weight loss programs*, aids in elimination*, contains antioxidants*. Yerba Mate is more than 'just' a tea, it's a power house!

This is a great alternative to coffee or any soda product and a great way to start your day. Yerba Mate is high in caffeine which is the good caffeine expressed from the tea leaf. Yerba Mate is a great source of anti-oxidants as well. Drinking 3 to 5 cups of this a day will keep you energized and lessen your need to snack on un- healthy items. However, I do believe in snacking throughout the day on raw foods such as carrots, celery, nuts, raw cacao chocolate and lots of sprouts. Again I cannot stress the importance of getting away from sodas, especially diet sodas. There is nothing diet about it, except of course for the word "die" (you will slowly 'die' if you drink 'it'!) Sodas have absolutely no nutritional value. The aspartame in diet drinks is deadly. Take a look at the sweetest deception chapter to learn about this deadly toxin. Aspartame is notorious for sinus infections, migraines and high blood sugar levels. It is also linked to onset of diabetes and stresses the adrenals.

If you cannot start drinking Yerba Mate right away, then start with a green or white tea, preferably organic teas, not some generic brand or some big corporation. Try HerbEscent Herbal teas. These are amazing health teas made by one lady known as the 'Medicine Lady'. Check her out on this site www.herbescentorganics.com I incorporate these teas every day as well. There is something for everyone here. Having too much tea is like having too much fun! You just can't have enough of the good stuff.

Here are some other great drinks you can also enjoy via Guayaki company. These are great alternatives to those "energy" drinks or shots. These are energetic alright, but in a very healthy way. So look for your natural energy in your local health food store today!

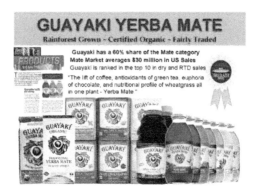

Photo taken from the Guayaki web site

The processing and picking of tea leaves are an essential part of how tea is effective. Herbal teas are extremely good for you. It is recommended that you drink 5 cups of tea per day to keep healthy metabolism and good anti-oxidants in the body. Drinking teas high in natural caffeine and anti-oxidants help improve the metabolism and enable you to digest your food better. Also take note that drinking herbal teas will reduce the risk of heart attack, stroke and some cancers. It has also been shown to boost the immune system and protect bones. Drinking green tea has also been known to improve cholesterol levels and protect the liver. As you can see there are many benefits to drinking tea. Yogi brand makes an excellent variety of teas as well. www.yogiproducts.com   There are many other health drinks on the market such as Bragg's Apple Cider Vinegar drinks, Aloe Drinks, and Kombucha. Ahh, the power of Kombucha to get the body FUELED for the day. The best drinks are obviously the ones you make yourself, so you know what is in it. But for those of you who claim to have no time, then the above mentioned companies are certainly ones to give a try.

Keeping yourself in optimum health will help you with fat burning metabolism. Tea is a cheap convenient way to remedy a weakened system. It is best to drink your tea hot or at room temperature. In fact, it is best to drink any drink at room temperature or hot. Why? Because this helps dissolve the fats from food you have just eaten to be more easily expelled from your body. What happens to butter, oil or meat fat when put in an ice cold glass of water? It solidifies. Did you know that America has one of the highest rates of heart attacks and heart disease? Remember we just realized that when, butter, oil or any fat from meat is put in cold water it solidifies. So it only makes sense that when you drink your ice cold drink with lunch or dinner, your arteries and intestines will get clogged because of the coldness being poured over the butter or fats you have just consumed. This makes it extremely difficult for your body to digest your foods. So if your drink is body temperature or hot, then the fatty foods will not be able to solidify, therefore enabling the fats and oils to be dissolved and more easily able to pass through your intestine.

This is just a thought to ponder. A very good thought to take heed to as well. Americans want that 'cold, quenching thirst' kind of feeling. Americans love their drinks cold and with ice.

Actually the opposite should be done. When drinking room temperature drinks, you will not have that 'dying of thirst' feeling. Also if you add lime or lemon to your water, this aids in hydration and quenches your thirst. Try it. Very important to stay well hydrated during the day.

Of course water, we can't forget about this magnificent wonder, is very beneficial for your well-being. It is best to drink 4 glasses of purified water daily. The rest can be tea or organic drinks. Water also helps our bodies to detoxify naturally. Keep in mind to drink only purified very clean, mineralized and filtered water.

Have you checked out what's in your water lately? As you know, our water supply is very polluted. Ironically the pollution you are thinking about is not the worst enemy.   The pollution most water is contaminated with is chlorine, fluoride and "added minerals" for taste. Added minerals for taste? What is that? Who knows what they put in it. Water in the pure state taste amazing and needs no 'added minerals' as fresh pure water has the earth's minerals of it's own. There are still plenty of sources to get clean water from. There are many springs throughout the world and the United States as well. If you do not have access to one of God's beauties and cleansers of the earth, then you would be doing well to invest in a good filtering system for your home. Making sure the filter takes both the chlorine and fluoride out of the water leaving you with the best of nature's minerals. The food industry and

USDA tell consumers it is safe to have chlorine in your drinking water as this helps to kill any bacteria. Would you pour yourself a glass of your pool water? Of course not! Speaking of pool water, it is really a bad idea to have chlorine as your disinfectant agent in the water as your skin is the largest organ of the human body. Therefore, it will absorb more of the chlorine than if you were drinking it. Use or invest in a salt water pool, or use baking soda to disinfect and balance the ph levels of the pool. Remember, one of my philosophies is, if you can't eat it then don't put it on your skin! Of course the USDA says chlorine in small amounts will not harm you. While this could be true if only ingested once in a life time or once per year, but how many 'small' amounts will one consume in one day?

Chlorine, a necessary disinfectant used to kill harmful, disease-causing bacteria. Unfortunately, chlorine combines easily with other chemicals and naturally occurring organic material to form many carcinogenic substances. An example of this is trihalomethanes (THMs), which are associated with rectal, bladder and pancreatic cancers, and may cause damage to the nervous system. Chlorine has also been linked to heart attacks, strokes, premature senility and sexual impotency. When you think about it, the purpose of chlorine is to kill living organisms; as far as I know we are all living organisms! Even in small amounts, taken daily this poison builds up in our systems and causes harm. Chlorine has also been linked to skin disorders such as psoriasis, eczema and acne. It is also known to hinder weight loss and even promote weight gain. I know, I have been a testimony of this while living in New York for a few months with my husband. Yes, I always take my drinking portable water filter with me, however, because I am on the road so much I don't always carry my shower filter with me. While in New York, my legs started to constantly itch and then I noticed that I started getting bloated and my hands were beginning to swell. Wow, me, Mrs. Organic Guru having issues? Well, it totally slipped my mind that I was bathing in an unfiltered shower! Good grief! Sure enough, once I got to my refuge of purified water for my shower, my ailments cleared up in 2 weeks. Needless to say, chlorine is not for human consumption. Google the pros and the cons on this, then you make the decision to consume or not to consume, to bathe or not to bathe in it.

As for fluoride, this is a controversial topic. However, fluoride is NOT for human consumption. We will dig further into this topic in future books. Although I do believe that one should NEVER consume fluoride. Let's just say fluoride was good for prevention of cavities and to ease sensitive teeth. Ok, then peroxide is great for fighting infections and does wonders on whitening teeth and ridding gum infections. However it can be deadly if you swallowed a mouth full. There is however, food grade peroxide you can get to avoid the harm if accidentally swallowed. You tell me, do you want to drink fluoride? Not me, thank you.

Go into your bathroom and grab any tube of toothpaste. If it is a tube of fluoride toothpaste (as the vast majority are) it will, by law, have this warning printed somewhere on the tube or box: "If you accidentally swallow more than used for brushing, seek professional help or contact a poison control center immediately." In this case, "professional help" likely means a physician or a local ER, and "poison control center" essentially means start praying because you (or your child) just swallowed a bunch of poison.

Wait a minute? If fluoride were poison why would it remain a key ingredient in toothpaste, a dental hygiene product we put in our mouth every day? And isn't our municipal water supply teeming with fluoride? Fluoride remains in our water supply and despite the risk of fluoride poisoning; it remains a key ingredient in toothpaste, as well as an inert ingredient in soda, tea, diet pills and bottled water (basically, anything with water in it likely has fluoride).   Read   more: http://www.care2.com/greenliving/the-dark-truth-about-fluoride.html#ixzz2DaSMyBoy

The only way to be assured to get purified water you can trust is to filter it yourself. You can get an inexpensive filter that takes out such corrosion from your local health food store. I highly recommend getting one of these. Get one for drinking water and for showering. Remember, your skin is the largest organ. Therefore, it absorbs many more toxins which penetrate through the blood stream. I stress the importance of filtering systems due to the ongoing toxins you accumulate in your body. If your skin is the largest organ and absorbs more toxins than ingesting, then it only makes sense to STOP the accumulation of toxins. This alone will result in increased health and more glowing and radiant looking skin. Therefore, to have optimum health, skin and weight...it is very important to look at all the aspects of your daily toxin consumption.

I will give more details about our water deception and what is causing you a lot of sickness in the following book: 'What Does Our Creator Say About Our Food & Health'.

For those of you on the go, a great source to get an economically great filter product is www.nikken.com/prosperity4u . This is the one I use and carry with me on my tours across the nation. For all your water filter and wellness home needs. They have just what you need for on the go with their Sport Pi Mag® purification bottle, Travel Pi Mag® or at home for drinking, get the Pi Mag Aqua Pour purification. These are great to get you started on your way to very clean water. The Nikken Aqua Pour filtering system is one of the best I have found for a fraction of the cost. It not only takes out the chlorine and fluoride, but removes any and all harmful bacteria such as e-coli. Plus, this unique system has mineral rocks which put back in the essential minerals of magnesium, zeolite and calcium that other filter systems leave out therefore leaving the water dead. The Aqua Pour gives you living water. I will go into greater detail in the following book about the importance of fresh, clean water and ridding your water of all toxins while at the same time keeping all beneficial minerals that water gives you. There are entire house filtering systems to bathe in. As I told you, your skin is the largest organ on your body, therefore absorbing many more toxins than actually ingesting them. This is another way that toxins affect the thyroid and other vital organs, by sneaking in through your skin. This is also why it is equally important to evaluate the products you put on your skin such as lotions, skin care products and make up. Think about it, you are absorbing heavy toxins through your skin. So my philosophy is, 'if you would not put it IN your body, then why put it ON your body'?

Drinking matters are what really matters. Make it pure, make it alive and make water your drinking habit.

The Sweetest Deception

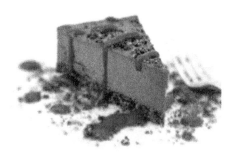

Photo, compliments of Navitas Naturals.

Sugar should be considered an illegal drug! White processed sugar that is. Sugar was never white it does not grow white in the cane. Sugar is brown. Sugar becomes white when the food industry bleaches, using bleaching agents like lime or carbon dioxide to whiten the sugar then it is chlorinated and refined. To make sugar white, sulfur dioxide may be bubbled through the cane juice before evaporation; this chemical bleaches many color-forming impurities into colorless ones. In sugar refining, raw sugar is further purified. It is first mixed with heavy syrup and then centrifuged clean. This process is called 'affination'; its purpose is to wash away the outer coating of the raw sugar crystals, which is less pure than the crystal interior. Refining and bleaching the sugar depletes any nutritional value the cane juice would have such as magnesium, potassium and even Vit. A and iron.

White sugar is the underlying cause in almost any disease, especially cancer. White sugar is notorious for hypoglycemia and causes candida overgrowth which causes cancer. White sugar also causes you to crave more bad sugar and starches. Oh how the food industry and FDA love this fact. Imagine, all the nation on a sugar craving binge for years. Though this sugar addiction wreaks havoc on the victim consuming it, it sure does pad the wallets of our big brother and big pharma! How does our sugar craving pad their wallets you ask? Well the more white sugar we consume, the more cancer risk and ADHD risk and diabetes problems we have. Not to mention obesity. So what happens? Well somebody has to "fix" these problems we encountered! Simply go to the doctor and get a drug which will 'hide' your ailments for a while, or take chemotherapy for the cancer you got from the sugar, because white sugar in the body is the breeding ground for cancer. Ah, and the wonderful cycle of the drug infested world begins. Remember, the best way to a person's heart is through their TUMMY! You better believe it. Oh, but it taste so good you say. Well of course! That's why it's the *sweetest deception.* "Oh, the better to treat your ailments with, my pretties"!

Let me remind you, erase everything you have been taught or have believed about foods and toxins. Again, we will discuss all this in future books. So take white processed sugar OUT of your pantry forever! The best thing you can do with this fake stuff is flush it down the toilet, literally! This is especially good if you have a septic tank as it will help grow beneficial bacteria to aid in breaking down waste.

Replace this white poison with sucanant. **Sucanat** sugar is dried sugar cane juice. Sucanat has a smaller proportion of sucrose, fewer calories and is loaded with vitamins and minerals. Sucanat sugar is filled with vitamins and minerals such as Potassium, Calcium, Magnesium, Vitamin A and many other nutrients. Sucanat retains its nutrient rich molasses substance. It has the least amount of paddling used to extract the molasses. It is made by crushing freshly cut sugar cane, extracting the juice and heating it in a large vat. Once the juice is reduced to a rich, dark syrup, it is hand-paddled. Hand paddling cools and dries the syrup, creating the dry porous granules that is called Sucanant. The word sucanant means: Sugar Cane Naturally. Nothing added, nothing taken out! Also it does not contain chemicals that take place during the refining process. The molasses is where you have the minerals, vitamins and fiber. This makes it a great substitute for brown sugar.

Turbinado is also great for your baking purposes. Turbinado comes from the first pressing of the sugar cane. It also contains 100 mg of potassium; 85 mg of calcium; 23 mg of magnesium; 3.9 mg of phosphorus; and 1.3 mg of iron.

You can also find much joy in the wonders of coconut palm sugar. This is also known as the 'sustainable' sugar. This sugar is my top choice for many recipes. Find your yummy treat recipe on my website. The coconut palm tree has long been used and appreciated for its edible resources by tropical communities. Among the most delicious parts of this plant is its sugar: the crystallized nectar of the coconut palm flowers, known as palm sugar. More than just lending a sweet taste, this sweetener is also extremely ecologically friendly: coconut palms produce an average of 50%-75% more sugar per acre than sugar cane, while using only a fifth of the resources. Coconut sugar contains calcium, magnesium, potassium, zinc, iron, copper, manganese, phosphorus and boron. Minerals are necessary for many body functions, such as muscle and bone growth, cell production, mental development and immune system and enzyme regulation. The glycemic index of coconut sugar is about 35 which is extremely low on the scale. It is also very high in amino acids which give it a great metabolic function. This is indeed the sugar of choice especially for diabetics. You can find more about this amazing wonder at www.navitasnaturals.com. Some excerpts taken from their page.

Other great and very clean sugars for the advanced organic and raw foodie are: medjool dates and maple syrup. Dates come from the 'Tree of Life' from Morroco and known as the 'dates of the kings'. The Medjool dates contain antioxidant flavonoids to help in the protection of cells and other body structures from the attack from oxygen free radicles. In doing so, it prevents the occurrence of lung, endometrial, prostate, colon, breast and pancreatic cancers. Maple syrup, PURE maple syrup not to be confused for 'pancake or waffle syrup', I'm talking about Grade B pure maple syrup alone. It has 54 known compounds that are known to have health benefits, making it especially appealing as a sweetener. It has also been discovered that pure maple syrup plays a role in lowering blood pressure therefore being a great 'sweetener' for diabetics. It has also been known for fighting cancer and bacterial illnesses due to its anti-oxidant and anti-inflammatory properties. So these two amazing natural pure sweeteners are what I highly recommend keeping in your kitchen pantry at all times!

If you must sweeten your tea or organic coffee, then do so safely. Stevia or Xylotol or Palm Sugar, these are the perfect alternatives to man-made sugar. Of course if you have any kind of cancers growing, you will want to avoid most sugars until you are free and clear of any tumors. With that being said, as per Dr. Patrick Vickers of the Gerson Treatment Hospital, natural earth made sugars play an important role in healing cancer patients. Sugars such as coconut, date, honey, fruit and brown rice syrup are helpful for cancer patients. For the record, did you know that consuming sugars in their natural state with-out the contamination from man, is completely safe and good for you to consume for a healthy balance. In fact, real natural sugars are even safe and recommended for cancer patients as suggested by Dr. Patrick Vickers of the Gerson Treatment Center. Before reading any further, please do not misinterpret this to implicate to consume as much sugar as you want. Keep in mind that consuming sugars in the natural state must be of the sugars listed in this book and never to be consumed in excess amounts.

Brown rice syrup is also one of the cleanest sugars to consume and is more diabetic friendly than even maple syrup. If you have cancer or know someone with cancer, please consult with Dr. Patrick Vickers founder of the Gerson Treatment Clinic. His number can be found in the back of this book. This way you are not misunderstanding my opinions about REAL NATURAL sugar consumption.

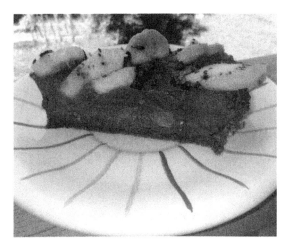

Lynnette's Raw Cacao Fruit Delight with Flax Crust

LOADED with Magnesium, Potassium, Zinc, Omegas, Protein, GREENS and Medium chain fatty acid and Anti-Oxidants.

RAW Cacao Fruited Delight

Crust:
1 cup Flax Meal
1/2 Cup Almond meal
1/2 Cup Coconut oil
1/4 Cup Brown rice syrup
1 tsp. Real Celtic Sea Salt
Blend well in vita mix and roll out in pie plate
Filling:
1/2 Cup Raw Cacao powder
2 heaping Tablespoons PHresh greens
1/2 cup Flax Meal
1/4 Cup Almond meal
1/2 Cup coconut oil
3/4 Cup cashew butter
1/4 Cup coconut sugar
1/4 cup cacao nibs
1 tsp Celtic Sea Salt
2 Tablespoons Moringa Powder
1 Avocado & 2 bananas

Blend well in Vita Mix till smooth. Pour into prepared pie crust. Top with Fruit of choice such as Banana and Kiwi! Set in Freezer to harden.

Eat and ENJOY this amazing healthy treat! Great for the kiddos. Especially if you can't get them to eat lunch or dinner, feed them this with NO guilt!

"Believe it or not, the real unadulterated sugars are what our bodies in fact need. When the body is acidic (build-up of hydrogen ions---hence PH----potential hydrogen) it cannot utilize oxygen properly. If it cannot use oxygen to metabolize sugars those sugars will fall into anaerobic glycolysis and will be converted into lactic acid instead of ATP. Cancer feeds on lactic acid so sugar is not the culprit in cancer. It is the body's inability to utilize and breakdown sugar. That is the problem! You must create the proper cellular environment to achieve that. An alkaline diet and absolutely no added sodium will prevent cellular edema. In that environment sugars can be metabolized properly. Our patients are getting 20 lbs. of fruit and veggie sugars daily, so how can it be that we are reversing advanced cancer? That is why".

Dr. Patrick Vickers

SweetLeaf Stevia® is the brand I use. Stevia leaves were introduced to Europe, in 1899, by a South American naturalist, Moses S. Bertoni. The Guarani Indians of Paraguay have been known to use the herb for a period of 1,500 years. This herb is a remarkable substitute for sugar, due to its non-synthetic and zero-calorific values. Stevia or *Stevia rebaudiana* is undoubtedly the big player, when it comes to alternative sweeteners. According to the World Health Organization (WHO), stevia has such sweet compounds which do not have any carcinogenic activity. Stevia contains most of the essential minerals and vitamins required for good health. Stevia has been known for its health benefits, for a long time. Best of all, Stevia gives you a feeling of even energy, rather than the ups and downs created with white sugar.

Believe it or not, the FDA in the United States has approved the usage of Stevia, not as a sweetener, but as a "dietary supplement" that helps balance blood sugar and blood pressure! At first the FDA reversed it's approval of Stevia being imported from Paraguay due to the pressures of other artificial sweetener companies. Hmmm, imagine that! For more information on this story, go to www.sweetleaf.com
There are virtually no calories in Stevia. You can bake with Stevia since the extracts are heat stable. SweetLeaf Stevia® is the trusted brand I use.
Do not be confused with the brand Truvia. Truvia is made from the Coca-cola and Cargill (the large agri giant) companies. They embarked on the wonderful benefits of stevia. One can patent an artificial food. Real herbs and foods cannot be patented. Truvia does have some part of the stevia plant in it, but it also has "other" ingredients that are detrimental to one's health. Truvia can be patented because they are not 100% stevia extract. The first listed ingredient is Erythritol (a naturally fermented sugar

alcohol), and Rebiana (which is the extraction of the actual sweet part of the plant) as well as other "natural flavors." While rebiana does not have any adverse effects on a person, it is the 'refining' process that is dangerous to one's health. So when you refine the natural sweet extract and then mix with fermented sugar, you are destined to have ailments. Excessive consumption of Erythritol (over 80 grams per day) may result in digestive upset, diarrhea, and bloating. Another reason the FDA 'approved' stevia as a "sweetener" for Truvia is due to the pressure of the giants Coca-cola and Cargill. You might also take note that the stevia crops that Cargill uses are from China!

Read more about this story on the link below:
http://www.healthynewage.com/blog/stevia-fda-approved/#ixzz18LIifuzZ

Guess how many ingredients stevia has? One! Yep, you don't need anything to make stevia as it is a plant all its' own. I grow this plant for my family and use it's wonderful leaves to sweeten my drinks. Stevia is a great alternative for diabetics. Do not use splenda or any other fake sweeteners listed under aspartame.

Here is a little factual information about our friend aspartame.

Equal, Nutrasweet, Equal Measure, Spoonful, Canderal (E951)

Aspartame was not approved until 1981, in dry foods. For over eight years, the FDA refused to approve it because of the seizures and brain tumors this drug produced in lab animals. The FDA continued to refuse to approve it until President Reagan took office (a friend of Searle) and fired the FDA Commissioner who wouldn't approve it. Dr. Arthur Hull Hayes was appointed as commissioner. Even then, there was so much opposition to approval, that a Board of Inquiry was set up. The Board said: "Do not approve aspartame." Dr. Hayes overruled his own Board of Inquiry.

Shortly after Commissioner Arthur Hull Hayes, Jr., approved the use of aspartame in carbonated beverages, he left for a position with G.D. Searle's Public Relations firm.

Long-term Damage

Aspartame appears to cause slow, silent damage in those unfortunate enough to not have immediate reactions and a reason to avoid it. It may take one year, five years, 10 years, or 40 years, but it seems to cause some reversible and some irreversible changes in health over long-term use.

Aspartame disease mimics symptoms or worsens the following diseases

fibromyalgia, arthritis, multiple sclerosis (MS), Parkinson's disease, lupus, multiple chemical sensitivities (MCS), diabetes and diabetic complications, epilepsy, Alzheimer's disease, birth defects, chronic fatigue syndrome, lymphoma, lyme disease, attention deficit disorder (ADD), panic disorder, depression and other psychological disorders

*A common ploy from Monsanto is to claim that aspartame is "safe" yet a few select people may have "allergic" reactions to it. This is typical Monsanto nonsense, of course. Their own research shows that it does not cause "allergic" reactions. It is there way of trying to minimize and hide the huge numbers of toxicity reactions and damage that people are experiencing from the long-term use of aspartame.

Remember, Monsanto is regulated by the FDA (food and death administration) in which Monsanto's own Michael Taylor is head of the FDA. You tell me, what sense does this make?

How it happens

Methanol, from aspartame, is released in the small intestine when the methyl group of aspartame encounters the enzyme chymotrypsin (Stegink 1984, page 143). Free methanol begins to form in liquid aspartame-containing products at temperatures above 86 degrees F also within the human body.

The methanol is then converted to formaldehyde. The formaldehyde converts to formic acid, ant sting poison. Toxic formic acid is used as an activator to strip epoxy and urethane coatings. Imagine what it does to your tissues!

*****These findings taken from Organic Consumers Association and www.dorway.com

For those of you who are bent on using Splenda as your alternative sweetener of choice, you may want to consider this first. Splenda is the brand name for sucralose and it was invented by accident when scientists were formulating an INSECTICIDE. Yikes! Somehow, I do not know how or why, they had a taste of their formulation and realized it tasted 'sweet'. So the ingredients that were to become an insecticide, are now presented to you for your sweet tooth and drinking pleasure. So indulge yourselves my friends as you may just rid your system of a few "bugs" and a lot more things as well! Don't take my word for it, go to this website and read the full story. http://www.brighthub.com/health/diet-nutrition/articles/31518.aspx

Read the article near the end of the book to get facts on aspartame and splenda.

Honey is great as well. Use local honey in the county you live as this is best to better help prevent and fight allergies. Of course if you are diabetic, then it is best to use only stevia or the pure maple syrup (which can lower blood sugars) or medjool date or no sweetener at all. In my following books, I will talk about how to prevent and remedy diabetes. Maple syrup and date sugars are very clean natural sweeteners to use at any time. But do NOT substitute maple syrup or honey for the very well marketed MYTH of Agave. Why? Agave has had an awesome marketing campaign to lead the public that this is the "new honey" or "natural sweetener". What they fail to tell you is that it has been processed using high heating methods. This causes the nectar to have a chemical change and therefore reacts the same way as high fructose corn syrup. The only way agave nectar is good for you at all is only if the nectar is cold pressed extracted and you KNOW where the plant came from. Most companies do not do this, so it is best to leave this nectar alone unless you can track the plant and extraction method and the place it came from.

You will note, I do promote sweet treats. I do not deprive myself of sweet indulgences. Oh, so satisfying! I just encourage you to use caution and knowledge when eating sweets. Know the facts, know the sources. You can 'clean up' any house hold recipe. Just simply make the change to real foods instead of the fake stuff! I have some great recipes of my own as well as I have a great friend, Liana Werner-Gray, author of The Earth Diet, who has an amazing recipe book. You can find her information in the back of this book. *'Fuel for the Body with The Earth Diet'* recipes.

Oh, the wonders of our beloved CHOCOLATE! I am talking RAW Cacao chocolate. Not to be confused with cocoa. Completely different processes.

Yes, I say have your cake and eat it too! Can you imagine never depriving yourself of those sweet indulgences again? Can you imagine chocolate cake that's actually good for you? I have those amazing recipes for you.

Raw cacao has the highest antioxidant value of all the natural foods in the world! That's what I'm talking about. Don't get Raw Cacao mixed up with 'chocolate', 'candy' or milk chocolate. Also do not confuse it with 'cocoa'. These are NOT the same as the cacao bean.

The official scientific name of the cacao tree is Theobroma Cacao. "Theobroma" is Latin for "food of the gods". Cacao is pronounced "ka-COW". The words "cacao" and the more commonly used term "cocoa" both refer to the cacao bean, the seed of the Theobroma Cacao fruit. So YES, cacao chocolate seed is actually a fruit!

Cacao beans are one of the most nutrient rich and complex foods known to man. Cacao is considered by some experts to be the antioxidant food and to have #1 source of magnesium of any food. Nutrients and Minerals Found in Cacao are: Magnesium, Iron, Chromium, Anandamide "The Bliss Chemical", Theobromine, Antioxidant Flavonoids, Manganese, Zinc, Copper, Omega 6 Fatty Acids, Phenethylamine (PEA), Tryptophan, Serotonin, Endorphins, Sulfur, Calcium, Potassium, N-acylethanolamines, Oleic Acid, Heart-Healthy Monounsaturated Fat, MAO Inhibitors.

Historically, cacao has been used to treat everything from kidney disorders and liver disease to depression and tickly coughs, but scientists now believe the antioxidants in it could also help prevent cancers and heart disease, and increase blood flow to the brain, fighting dementia into the bargain.

BENEFITS OF CACAO Nutrients and Minerals

1. *Reduces appetite and helps in weight loss*

2. *Helps with cardiovascular health*

3. *Lowers LDL Cholesterol*

4. *Reduces the Risk of Stroke and Risk of Heart Attacks*

5. *Helps to Protect from Environmental and Metabolic Toxins*

6. *Acts as an Anti-Depressant and Balances the Mood*

7. *Balances the Brain Chemistry*

8. *Helps to Reduce PMS Systems*

> 9. *Helps to Increase Focus and Alertness*
>
> 10. *Builds Strong Nails and Hair*
>
> 11. *Detoxifies the Liver*
>
> 12. *Helps with Healthy Pancreas Functioning*
>
> 13. *Balances Blood Sugar*
>
> 14. *Helps to Fight Cavities*
>
> 15. *Builds a Stress Defense Shield*
>
> 16. *Facilitates Anti-Aging and Rejuvenation*

What a super healthy fruit. Yes, that's right cacao is actually a FRUIT - and it is actually one of the most healthy fruits commonly eaten by man! ***some excerpts taken from the www.survivalmonkey.com and www.navitasnaturals.com*

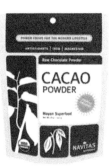

You just can't get much better than that! Remember to always make it RAW cacao and organic and as dark as possible. None of this Hershey, dove, or candy stuff! Toxic FREE food is the KEY to health, weight loss, ultimate sex and radiant skin.

Navitas Naturals Cacao Powder brings the chocolate factory to your kitchen. It instantly transforms smoothies, desserts, pies, and countless other recipes into the healthiest chocolate indulgence around. Put a spoonful into your next treat and understand why this super food has been enjoyed for thousands of years. Plus, with no added sugar, Navitas Naturals Cacao Powder is an exceptionally healthy way to stock up on antioxidants and important minerals like magnesium and iron. Check out the cacao recipe section for great ideas, and make your life as chocolatey as you please! I always have my chocolate and eat it too! A raw chocolate treat a day can keep the doctor away! Try my amazing chocolate ball recipe. Quick, easy and delish!

RAW VEGAN CHOCOLATE COCONUT BALLS

1/2 C. Coconut BUTTER NOT oil
4 TBL Honey or Brown Rice syrup
1 TBL Coconut OIL
1 TBL Brown Sugar
2 TBL. Coconut Milk
1 TBL Almond Extract
8 TBL RAW Cacao Powder
2 TBL Cacao Nibs
4 TBL Hemp Hearts
Coconut Shreds or Hemp Hearts to roll balls in.

Mix all together very well except for coconut shreds. Make small balls and roll them into the coconut shreds or hemp hearts. Place in freezer for 10 minutes. Then keep in freezer or fridge and enjoy anytime for a HEALTHY snack!

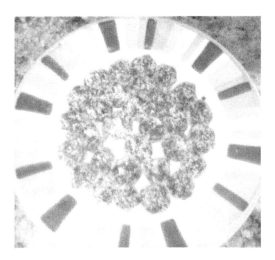

Here is also another amazing quick and easy recipe I keep on hand at all times. I make this weekly and keep it in the freezer for quick snacking. My amazing Cacao Bark recipes. You can use almonds, cashews, coconut flakes, cacao nibs, etc. for this recipe.

ALMOST RAW CACAO BARK

4 oz. Coconut Butter

4 Tbl. Coconut Oil

6 Tbl. Cacao Powder

½ Cup Coconut Sugar

½ Cup Almond or Flax Meal

½ Cup Sliced Almonds, cashews, coconut flakes or etc.

½ Cup Cacao Nibs

1 Tsp. Almond extract

1 Tsp. Celtic Sea Salt

Heat on very low heat to melt coconut butter, coconut oil and coconut sugar until dissolved. Continue heating on low heat and mix in almond or flax meal, stirring continually. Then mix in remaining ingredients. Pour onto non-bleached waxed paper covered cookie sheet. Place in freezer. Break into wedges, eat, enjoy!

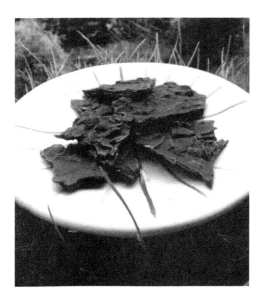

Remember to follow me on face book to stay up to date on the new books and my seminars and locations by searching for fuel for the body bike tour in the search bar. There you will find daily health tips, smoothie recipes and what is going on in the food industry and the media. This is a great way to keep up with our amazing bicycle tours across the nation as well. We tour across the country to educate the world about organic and toxic free living. Our desire is to become a healthy nation to have a clean planet for generations to come. Let's make a pledge to maintain our food and health freedoms.

The below picture is NOT what we want to become. We see beauty, abundance, love and prosperity in our near future.

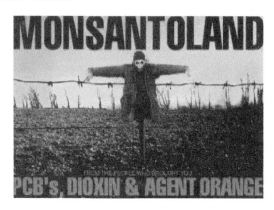

Photo taken from the Organic Consumers Association web page

Are you a 'Salt Phobia'?

Speaking of white stuff and refining and bleaching, do you know the truth about salt? We are salt phobias in America. We avoid salt like the plague! In fact, we are told to consume very little salt or no salt at all.

I lived without salt in my diet for several years due to my kidney surgery at the ripe young age of 8 years old. I was told to always avoid salt as it would cause complications to my kidneys and make my legs swell and other ailments to my body. Well that was and is true, true to the fact that 'fake' salt would do this to me. Yes, once again, the food industry and big pharma has lied to us! Of course, salt the way the food industry refines and bleaches it is very bad for us. This is the way of the elites' agenda. They say, let's make salt look "pretty" and pleasing to the eye by bleaching it. This way we can use any 'ole salt out there and it will be fine, because we will just bleach it white and "add" iodine back in it for the health benefit. Wink, wink! Then we tell the consumers they must avoid salt as this is detrimental to their health as they consume so much of it. After all we put it in all canned goods, processed foods and boxed items. So now it is off to ailment city for our unsuspecting victims as they have now destroyed their thyroid due to NO salt intake and the intake of the fake stuff!

Did you know that salt is NOT pure solid white either? Salt is 'snow white' when the food industry get their nasty hands on it. Salt in the pure form is pink, grayish green, black, brown and off white. There is one rare salt that looks to be pure white, but when one looks closely they will see the pinkish tint it has. This is Makai Pure salt. Makai Pure® Mineral-rich sea water is extracted from 2,000 feet below the surface of the Pacific Ocean and remains untouched and pure through its transformation into Makai   Pure®   Gourmet   Sea   Salt. Scientists have found that deep sea currents are the coldest, saltiest waters and do not readily mix into other ocean water. Celtic Sea Salt® Makai Pure® is absolutely nothing other than the extracted pure minerals from the deep, which crystallize in a pharmaceutical grade facility. (this paragraph on Makai Pure® taken from www.selinanaturally.com).

Salt is actually very beneficial to the body. Again, God put plenty of salt on this earth for a reason...to benefit us!

I tell you all of this because I know the benefit of real salt. Up until 9 years ago, I was still having all sorts of swelling in my legs and continued to have complications with my kidneys year after year with hospital and emergency room visits. I was put on all kinds of water pills, fluid pills and kidney pills. It wasn't until I learned from my son's doctor, who cured   him   of   his   Recurrent   Respiratory Papillomatosis (RRP) disease, the difference between real and fake salts. This is where I was convinced that consuming real salt would have a positive impact on my kidney health. What? No way! I then began studying the benefits of salt and salt in the real form. Wow, amazing! I then found Celtic Sea Salt® and studied this amazing mineral. I then started adding this Celtic Sea Salt® to my diet on a daily basis and behold, as if magic, my fluid started diminishing from my legs. Oh what joy, I now had ankles! I never saw my ankle bone. You have to excuse me while I get a bit excited about having ankles. If you would have only seen my legs/ankles. I had none. We just deemed it was due to cheerleading and constant workout on my legs and I just had thick skin. Right! Imagine, I could now consume salt and enjoy life. It was the horrific chlorine and refining of salt that destroyed my system. Real salt, such as Celtic Sea Salt® has tremendous healing virtues. This salt actually aids in fluid elimination, mucus elimination and normalizes blood pressure. In fact, I mix 1/4 teaspoon of 'real' salt with 3 - 8 ounces of purified warm water and drink nightly! Who would have thought, I am drinking salt water and my kidney problems are gone and I am healthier than ever!

Now, I do not advise for everyone to consume this amount of salt on a daily basis. The recommended daily amount of real salt to consume is about 1/8 to ¼ teaspoon Celtic or Himalayan salt to 32 oz. purified water. Please check with your natural practicing health care provider before consuming salt as I do.

**A special note, if you have cancer or you know someone with cancer, please do not consume salt until directed by a natural health care provider. If you are on the Gerson Treatment, the Gerson Therapy protocol exercises NO SALT, period, for their cancer patients or patients with severe medical conditions.

Celtic Sea Salt® has 84 trace minerals such as magnesium, zinc, iron, potassium and sodium which provide the necessary nutrients and protect the body from the harshness of sodium chloride that we consume from commercial salt. The appropriate magnesium content ensures that unused sodium is quickly and completely eliminated from the body through the kidneys to prevent harm. Celtic Sea Salt® is a grayish green moist salt that is ideal for soups or garnish. It is safe to consume ¼ to ½ teaspoon or more of this salt just plain in 32 oz. of warm water on a daily basis along with using it for cooking and garnishing. Again, I would encourage you to seek the advice from your natural health care provider. I use this method of consuming real salt for my kidney health. For kidney patients, I highly recommend an amazing kidney doctor who helps patients around the world reverse their most advanced kidney disorders. You can find her at: www.theholistic-kidney.com

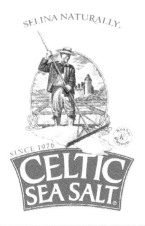

"*Selina Naturally® Deep Sea Salt is an exceptional product I discovered a few years ago. I thought I had seen the best until I found this one. It is a great finishing salt for salads and fruits. The potassium is higher than any other salt on the mark.*

I use my Celtic Sea Salt® brand for baking and cooking and the Deep Sea Salt as a finishing salt. The flavor of both is amazing!

Being in the business for over 30 years, I have had the opportunity to observe the changes that this necessary ingredient, salt, has gone through. I have also had the opportunity to explore salts from all over the world in order to continue the sourcing of high mineral, lower sodium chloride sea salts. Given my personal

107

relationships I have with the harvesters, I am confident in my ability to assure the consumer of mineral balance and quality control.

God meant for us to eat salt with a natural balance of potassium, sodium chloride and magnesium. This is why we feel so good when we consume the minerals of sea salts vs. common table salt. We welcome any questions you may have regarding salt and the role it plays on the body. Visit us online at www.SelinaNaturally.com for additional information, resources and products"!

Selina DeLangre
CEO / Founder of Celtic Sea Salt

Of course there are more 'real' salts you can purchase just as Selina described above. In my opinion, this is the best salt in the sea.

In my opinion, Himalayan salt is the best salt on earth. Himalayan salt is a pink to amber color. This salt comes straight from the Himalayan Mountains and boast over 94 trace essential minerals. This salt produces negative ions for your body to off-set the positive ions your body produces. The combination of positive and negative ions are a great way to achieve equal energy balance for your cells. This is also a great way to boost the immune system.

Himalayan salt also helps with allergies and fluid retention. Use this amazing salt for bath soaks or you can even purchase Himalayan salt stones. These are perfect for massages or exfoliating in the shower. Have you seen those beautiful Himalayan salt lamps? Yes, these are pure salt and when heated these also produce the negative ions a person needs. These lamps are ideal for asthma, ADHD and anxiety. Try one today. Put a salt lamp in every room. If asthmatic especially keep one in the room at all times. Also, great for autistic children, it helps them to relax. If you keep those Himalayan salt rocks near the pillow for them to massage at night, it helps to soothe the mind. See www.phreshproducts.com for all details on this Himalayan gem.

I personally use the different real salts every day. I alternate the salts into my diet. I do use the salt lamps and the salt stones for massages and keep one in the shower for exfoliation as well as salt mineral absorbing.

So you see, another misguided path we have been led down through the years. Truth: Pure, bleached table salt is BAD. Real un-refined God given salt is GOOD! Look around you, why do we have an abundance of God's great mineral on this planet? It is one of the best preservatives ever as well.

When man tries to diminish, take away or add to God's word, it leads to 'Spiritual' weakness and spiritual sickness. The same rule can be applied to food. When man adds to or strips 'real' food of its nutrients, it will lead to physical sickness and ailments.

> *"The better you take care of your body, the better it will take care of you."* L. Marie

Food is often a picture of God's word. Man thinks he can 'improve upon God's truth just as man thinks he can 'improve' upon what God made edible. Just giving you a little 'food for thought' here. I will go into more detail about eating what the Creator gave us to eat in book 3: *"What Does Our Creator Have to Say About Our Food and Health"*? Stay tuned for that informative and inspiring book.

**Please ask your natural healthcare provider on how much 'real' salt to consume before consuming.

The Secret Essential Food Staples

Ok, here it is, the *secret* to get you on your way to a healthier, happier more beautiful/handsome YOU! Guess what?   It really is not a secret.   Just information being brought to life for you! This book is a "jump start" if you will, to get your body programmed to eat more healthy and to slow those cravings of bad sugars and starches. This is really not a secret, unless you've never heard of these. These are staples to give you a 'jump start' to start living a life full of health and longevity. These foods are NOT the quick fix to your weight problem, they are simply enhancements for you to get on the right track. Incorporate these foods every day of your life and you will see and feel the difference. You will discover while reading this book and incorporating the foods and ideas I have given you, that it is NOT the calories, fat grams or points that matter, but rather the TOXINS that wreak havoc on your body.

*Remember when changing any part of your daily diet it is recommended you visit your health care provider. This ensures your health and safety.

You should look for these 3 essential foods. If you have trouble finding them, you can always order from my website. However, I want you to understand you can purchase these products at most health food stores.

1)   ORGANIC APPLE CIDER VINEGAR

with the 'MOTHER'. It has to have the mother otherwise you do yourself a great injustice and possibly a reverse effect. The 'mother' is the pure unadulterated whole fermented apple without ever being bleached, distilled or whatever the industry does to taint it. (My preferred choice is Bragg's brand)

2)   ORGANIC   EXTRA   VIRGIN COCONUT OIL   Must be Organic and Extra Virgin. Otherwise you will not get the great flavor, nor will you get the finest, purest first pressed and essential nutrients. (My preferred choice is Selina Naturally via Celtic Sea Salt brand.)

3)   ORGANIC HEMP SEED HEARTS Most hemp is generally organic since it requires no pesticides. Beware of some so called "hemp protein powders" out there, as some companies simply do not take the time

or care in processing the heart of the seed appropriately. Hence, it's nutritional value is lower as it has the shell ground up in it. (My preferred brand is Manitoba Harvest) So please take caution when getting these 'hemp protein powders' to be sure you have the nutrition levels to nourish your cells.

After you get these staples, this is what you do with them EVERYDAY! Then you will note additional MUST HAVE pantry staples for your healthy life style change.

1) As soon as you wake up in the morning, mix 3 - 4 teaspoons of Organic Apple Cider Vinegar w/the mother into 8 oz. water. (Yes, this is an acquired taste). Drink this as you take your natural and whole food vitamins. This enables your body to absorb the cider and helps with digestion, metabolism, and stomach problems and also helps aid in waste elimination. Also for more energy and a pick-me-up in late afternoon, you can mix this drink again. I prefer 3 Tbs. of ACV in 8 oz. water. Build yourself up to 3 tbl. For optimum results.

2) After you drink your cider vinegar, then eat 3 Tablespoons of Hemp Seed Hearts. These

are very tasty (like pine nuts). NOTE: for optimum results on weight loss, I recommend you eat these 3 Tbl. Plain with a spoon right before you eat your normal healthy breakfast. Then eat 2 more Tablespoons for lunch or before 2 p.m. You can eat these 2 plain again, or sprinkle on a salad, sushi, eggs, yogurt and etc. If you are doing this for healthy maintenance and not weight loss, then I recommend eating 3 Tablespoons per day. You can eat these plain or anyway you want, even in smoothies. Yummy!

3) Before you eat breakfast, eat 1 Tablespoon raw (yes raw) plain Organic Extra Virgin Coconut Oil. This helps to combat the bad fats you are about to consume. Do this for 5 days then increase to 2 times per day. Consuming 1 tablespoon before breakfast and then before lunch. After the next 5 days, increase again to 3 times per day. Consuming 1 tablespoon before breakfast, lunch and dinner. It is recommended to consume the coconut this slowly as to help your body get introduced to the high consumption of fat. Although very healthy for you, if you have not been used to this fat then your body may feel

overwhelmed. If your coconut oil solidifies and you have a hard time swallowing it, then let the jar sit in a hot pan of water to liquefy. This is easier for people to eat. I like mine either way. Never use a microwave to warm it!

OK...there you have it! The 3 Secret food staples and what to do with them. You should never be without these 3 foods in your home. These have just become your best friends and will always be by your side. You will eat these just like waking up and putting on your clothes. They are so tasty as well.

As I mentioned about the hemp seed hearts, you can consume them in the morning with breakfast and again with lunch or as a snack after lunch. Also continue eating as healthy as you can throughout the day, remembering to eat 6 times per day in very small portions.

Your typical daily intake of food will look something like this: breakfast, snack, lunch, snack, dinner then snack before bed.

**Please note, that if you have never cleansed or taken any detox tea, you may experience more waste elimination the first 2 days. Remember, a healthy person should have 2 to 4 bowel movements per day. This is a natural process to rid the body of toxin build up.   A healthy colon is a healthy & happy person!

If you do the mentioned 3 staple regimen and do NOTHING else, you WILL see a vast improvement of your cravings for bad starches and sugars, you will see reduced appetite and you will experience added energy. The only "side effect" you will experience is...weight loss! However, I do recommend taking more of the opinions I have and am about to give you. By taking the opinions I further give you will only enhance and help you see results faster.   By consuming these foods, your brain will be re-directed into wanting more of the 'good stuff'! Remember, these are NOT magic, nor quick fixes, but pure and simple SUPER HEALTH FOODS!

So basically what my typical daily routine consist of is this. I do everything I just told you with the 3 simple additions. I do eat breakfast each and every morning. Either eating oatmeal with hemp hearts and coconut sugar and coconut oil in it, or an egg frittata or fried egg in which I fry mine in coconut oil. Yummy! Then because I am constantly on the go go go, it is hard for me to juice every single day. I do recommend you doing a juice at least 3 times per week.   Some type of juicing is perfect for daily incorporation for optimum health. What I do is mix 1 teaspoon of the PHresh Greens into 1 8 oz shaker of water. The health benefits of this greens drink are amazing.   This company in no way promotes you substituting their greens for pure raw greens. However, they recommend you incorporating them as an additional way to get your greens. You actually get all your daily greens that is recommended in just 1 little teaspoon. These greens are RAW, non-irradiated and LIVING. The best pure greens I have found in my travels. You can also spritz the drink with a lime or you can even add chia seeds in the drink to really complete your cellular nutrition. I even incorporate these amazing greens into my to LIVE for chocolate vegan cake and brownies and my secret recipe PHresh Chocolate Balls. Find those recipes and many more on my website. Talk about yum and nutritional. See, I told you that to deprive yourself of treats is not in my vocabulary!   I will usually drink the greens drink sometime after breakfast as my hearty snack along with some raw fresh almonds or walnuts or a piece of my almond bark or phresh cacao balls. Next, I eat my lunch which consist of salad, raw veggies, or sautéed veggies. I will eat soups in the winter time and 2 to 3 times a month I do incorporate my red meat for my kidney health. More about meats in the following chapters. I will enjoy my freshly made hummus or yummy spring veggie rolls. Then I am always sipping on either Guayaki Yerba Mate or herbal teas through-out the day. Then for afternoon snack, I will have some fruit, such as an apple, blue berries, raspberries, kiwi or avocado. So many snacking choices when we eat toxic free. Then I have my dinner, which consist of quinea, couscous, veggies, occasional meat once or twice per month. I do try to practice the 85% raw diet. I also encourage you to at least start with 50% raw then slowly make your way to more raw foods daily. So many yummy foods can be consumed and yummy. This aids in better digestion and living foods going into a living body   Then before I head to bed, I always wind down with a cup of herbal tea. I also drink my diatomaceous earth water for the optimum amount of silica I can consume. Which, by the way, is great for hair skin and nails. I will also either enjoy a green apple with real salt sprinkled on it, or an avocado with cracked pepper sprinkled on it or even a nice bowl of granola with some coconut milk over it.

Keep in mind, I change my foods up daily to keep it fun and always get in season produce to nourish my body to the fullest extent. There are many choices us organic foodies have and not have to worry about gaining weight or getting sick or skin breaking out. See, food should be to LIVE for not to die for!

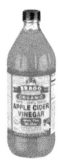

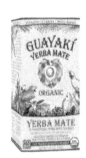

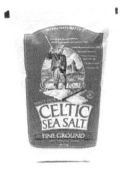

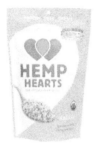
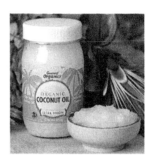

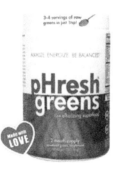

Pictured are the amazing super foods. I have also included the picture of Guayaki Yerba Mate as per the reference I made in drinking matters chapter as well as the Celtic Sea Salt and PHresh Greens, I mention for your daily routine. I Use these foods EVERY DAY! These are the food staples everyone should have stocked in their kitchen at all times!

Facts of the secret foods

Why these foods?

Now let's talk about why I chose these foods and why they are good for you and what each one does for the body.

Well, first of all, the American diet has been so restricted to fast foods, whether it be fast food restaurants or fast food out of a box. Americans are so impatient and want their food now. Our diet has turned in to a chemical warfare in our bodies. We have so many toxins in our bodies from the MSG, GMO and pesticide infested foods we eat and the pollution we breathe. In a world of "give me my food now and make it a biggie size", we have forgotten what real wholesome food taste like. Our bodies have been tormented and beaten down in a very slow way. Therefore, to change our bodies in a fast way would be impossible. You did not get out of shape over-night, so you will NOT get back into shape over-night. However, you can start detoxing your body immediately. Cleansing and purifying your body is a major part of weight control. You can do this with the 3 staples just given to you. Our bodies need to get rid of the toxin build up in the intestines. Ridding toxins of your body is so important for your well-being. Just think of years of pollution, chemicals, mono-sodium glutamate and genetically modified organisms being stored in your intestine. On average, the American public packs on 8 lbs. of toxins in their intestine each year. Ugh, how disgusting! This is all packed in tightly in the intestine preventing any form of rotation of the foods ingested. Wow, you harbor 8 lbs. of toxic build up in your colon? Imagine carrying this 8 lbs. and adding another 8 lbs. to it every year. Now granted, some of that, oh about 1 or 2 lbs. will be excreted. Just think, by cleansing your colon every year or every 6 months, you can lose 8 lbs. just like that! A healthy colon is a happy colon. Our bodies were meant to process food and eliminate waste. Do you think our bodies were meant for chemical consumption? Pesticide ingestion? Would you drink a bottle of fertilizer or insect repellant? Of course not! However, you are doing just that with our 'modern' American way of creating a chemical plant right in your kitchen pantry.

So the first step to a more regulated colon is to get those toxins out! Again, with the 3 staples you have just been given, this will be a small step to this toxin elimination. You can also start by drinking a detox tea. There are two inexpensive ones I recommend to start that are very easy to drink and taste good. Yogi brand Detox and Get Regular formulas. www.yogiproducts.com These teas come in a box of 16 tea bags. You simply drink this tea after your meal at lunch or dinner (or both). Even if you are out to dinner in the MSG infested world, you can take a tea bag with you and ask for a cup of hot water with lemon or honey. Just drink this tea with your meal and you can eliminate some of the toxins you just ingested.

Another great way to get those harmful toxins out of your system is by the use of a 'Far Infrared Sauna'. My top pick is Great Saunas. This company has mastered the benefits of a well built sauna to give you the maximum health benefits. Check out www.greatsaunas.com . We will discuss complete body cleansing and detoxing in the next book. Again, I do not want to overload your mind. This book is to keep it simple for you. Remember, we also discussed exploring the possibility of colonics I mention in the previous chapters. I highly encourage you to do this once per year, if you are an extremely clean eater, then get one every 2 years.

With all that being said, let's examine the 3 food staples.

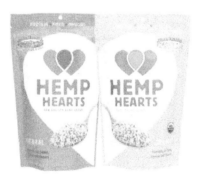

First we have Hemp Seed Hearts. Hemp Hearts are considered Nature's most Perfect Food.   Why? Hemp Hearts are the most concentrated source of essential nutrients known. Those who consume the amount listed previously, preferably with long fiber, raw vegetables & yogurt, notice that they have enough energy for the entire day. They also notice they will need to expel wastes after every meal and are not hungry again till mid-afternoon.

Hemp Hearts:

*Contains more required amino acids (proteins) than milk, meat or eggs.

*Is a complete protein source and more balanced than any soy product. (I discourage any soy products myself)

*Contains about 47% oil, 86% of is omega 3, 6 & 9. Omega 9's are lacking in our modern diet today, this is a very important omega to our digestive system as well as better fuel charge. It has much more of omega 3 than fish.

*Contains ALL the essential and Omega fats required for human health.

*Is suitable for those unable to consume gluten, sugar, milk, nuts or meat.

*Is perfect for people troubled with constipation.

*A 55 g serving (5 Tbl) contains 314 calories of energy from 20 g protein, 23.2 g unsaturated fats, 2.7 g saturated fats, 5.9 g carbohydrates, 3.3 g fiber, 2.6 mg iron, 40.6 mg calcium, 5 mg sodium, 5 mg vitamin e, .55 mg vitamin C, .07 mg vitamin B6, .18 mg vitamin B2, .76 mg vitamin B1, 1200 IU vitamin D, 2.2 IU vitamin A, .38 g Potassium, and .4 g Phosphorus.

As you can see, the Hemp Heart is loaded with POWER! Hemp fills the Brain instead of only the stomach. When your brain is full and satisfied, then your stomach doesn't yell at you. Your brain lets you know when to eat and how much to eat.

Also you will start to see an improvement in the texture of your skin and hair. The high omega content is excellent for more supple looking and feeling skin.

Again, I want to mention that Hemp Protein or Hemp Flour is not to be replaced for the actual hemp heart seed you can eat plain. Some companies make these products by grinding the wastes which remain after valuable oil has been extracted from whole hemp seeds. They are mostly composed of indigestible shells. So again, be aware of your sources when purchasing hemp flour or hemp protein powder. Manitoba Harvest, the brand I prefer, has the right technology for processing and making the protein powders and flours. Therefore, I do use their amazing chocolate hemp protein powder for that added snack for my day.

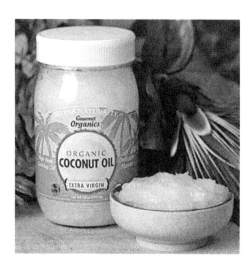

Ok, next we have Organic Extra Virgin Coconut Oil. Four thousand years ago, the early Ayurvedic practitioners discovered the health benefits of coconut oil. Despite western medicine belief, organic extra virgin coconut oil is the best oil in the world for you, both internally and externally! Oh how wonderful you skin will feel after slathering it all over. I love this stuff! Keep in mind that you must get the organic and extra virgin oil. This ensures you will be getting the first pressed of the coconut (just like the olive) and organic ensures that it has not been refined. Refining the coconut destroys it's natural antioxidants. Yes, coconut oil is high in saturated fat, 14 g per tablespoon full to be exact! Wow, this is taboo in the medical world. However, just like good cholesterol and bad cholesterol, there are good and bad fats. The lauric acid in the coconut oil is a good saturated fat. Coconut oil is made of mostly medium chain fatty acids, which are quickly converted to energy rather than stored as fat. These medium chain fatty acids actually attack the bad fats in your body, therefore allowing them to be eliminated more easily. The free fatty acids and monoglycerides in coconut oil help support the healthy functioning of the gastrointestinal tract by helping to maintain the healthy intestinal flora.

Organic Extra Virgin Coconut Oil:

*Helps maintain cholesterol levels that are already within the normal range

*Support the immune system

*Help maintain healthy intestinal flora

*Aids in weight loss

*Has anti-fungal and anti-bacterial properties which is great for skin irritations, burns and mouth sores

*Has NO cholesterol

*Has NO trans fatty acids

Coconut oil has 125 calories per 1 tbl, 14 g total fat in which 13 g of those are saturated fats, 0 grams sodium, 0 grams of protein and 0 grams of carbohydrates.

So now you understand that coconut oil is a great staple for every household. I also recommend cooking with coconut oil instead of the other oils you use. This oil has a very high smoke point and is a great way to eliminate the bad fats while you are cooking. Eggs are great scrambled in this oil as well as sautéed fish. You can also use coconut oil for baking cakes, muffins or breads. This makes for a very moist cake! This is another step in the nutritional direction of changing your eating habits. You can also add coconut oil to smoothies, the coconut oil will solidify because of any cold items you put in smoothie such as rice milk and frozen fruits. This is a great power boost for your smoothie, yummy! As I mentioned earlier, my preferred brand is Selina Naturally. This company has a long and reputable history of quality and purity. They understand how the coconut meat should be harvested. Founded by Selina DeLangre, with 30 years in the health industry avid health back ground. They not only have coconut oil, but they have the finest super foods in their product line.

Finally we have apple cider vinegar.

Apple Cider Vinegar with the 'Mother'

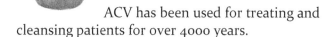

ACV has been used for treating and cleansing patients for over 4000 years.

The "Mother" in ACV is the whole un-adulterated fermented apple which has been aged in wood barrels. The 'mother' is the web like sediment that occurs at the bottom of the bottle. This is the most nutritional part of the vinegar as it has living enzymes which are vital to fighting infections and bacteria. It has not been distilled. It is best to shake the bottle slightly so that you always get parts of the mother when drinking. ACV is rich in enzymes and potassium (11 mg of potassium) and is a natural germ fighter. Great for fighting E Coli and other bacteria.

ACV also helps aid in digestion and is very good for irritable bowel syndrome. ACV also contains NO sugars. ACV is also great for cleansing of the arteries. There are many uses for apple cider vinegar such as making salad dressings, marinades and can also be used to treat the skin and scalp for dryness. Sure, many people have heard of the apple cider vinegar diet. However, this food alone will not give you the results you will see while incorporating all 3 items. Do not be deceived by plain apple cider vinegar. This may end up giving you the reverse effect as it contains no nutritional value and all the live enzymes have been removed due to distillation and heating. Raw apple cider vinegar with the 'mother' has never been heated. Bragg company (www.bragg.com) has perfected the 'mother' in ACV. They are a company with integrity and looks out for man's good health. Bragg's also has a great array of tinctures and amino acids. Also do not try to take a short cut in getting the apple cider vinegar capsules. These will have no benefit for you. Some people have said they can't stand the smell of ACV or even think about tasting it. Like I said, it is an acquired taste.

DO NOT TAKE SHORT CUTS! However, you CAN add a teaspoon of honey and some cinnamon to take the edge off.

A good philosophy to live by:

> *'If you continue cutting corners, you will soon be going only in circles'.*

As you can see, these 3 staples are very powerful healing foods. Used in conjunction with each other creates a great start to the cleansing process needed to have abundant health.

You won't want to miss out on my chapter of skin and hair care in the book following by using Braggs' ACV and Selina Naturally coconut oil.

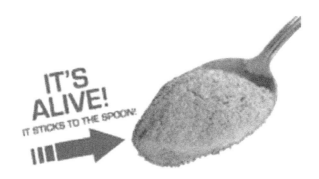

Next, my favorite addition to my daily routine is the PHresh Greens product. They are simply amazing! Why? Because the are RAW, living, non-irradiated and whole pure greens. Nothing else added in the ingredient list. Greens in its purest form in a container to be on the go with. As mentioned earlier, these are not meant to take the place of a well rounded salad or meal. They are simply an addition for your daily intake. However, if you just cannot get all the greens you need in one day, or you are on the road such as I am, then these are the perfect addition to take if you can't get that juice in. I even make vegan chocolate green cakes, vegan chocolate raw cacao balls, power pancakes and much more with these amazing super greens. Check website for recipes. But here is one for fun. Try these power pancakes.

Power Pancakes

1 & 1/2 C. Brown Rice Flour or Spelt
3 & 1/2 tsp. Bkg. powder
1 tsp. Soda,
2 Tbl. Phresh Greens
1 & 1/4 C. Coconut Milk
1 Egg
2 Tbl. HEMP Seed
1 tsp. Lemon juice or Apple Cider Vinegar

Mix well and pour onto hot Coconut Oiled skillet. Add blueberries for topping or into the mixture before cooking. Top also with HEMP Butter or coconut butter and drizzle with a little honey or dark maple syrup.

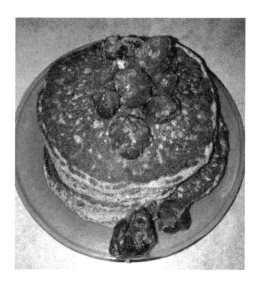

Benefits: Greens contain up to 70% Chlorophyll.*
Chlorophyll is the first product of light and contains
more light energy than any other element.*

Green drinks are high in oxygen like all green plants
that contain Chlorophyll. The brain and all body
tissues function at an optimal level in a highly
oxygenated environment.*

Green juice is a superior detoxification agent
compared to carrot juice and other fruits and
vegetables.*

pHresh greens® contains dehydrated juices and
powders from their organic ingredients. The
powders are made by first juicing the greens, and
then dehydrating them in low temperatures in order
to preserve the enzymes which helps retain its life
energy.*

Dr. Earp Thomas, associate of Ann Wigmore, says that 15 pounds of Wheatgrass is the equivalent of 350 pounds of carrots, lettuce, and celery and so on.*

**Excerpts taken from phreshproducts.com

Food can be fun and be your friend!

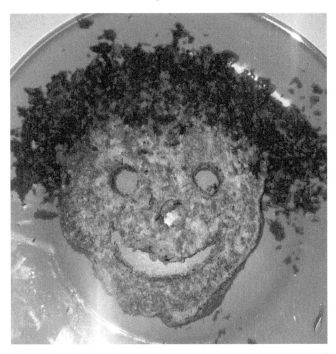

Lynnette's beet and carrot pancakes. Recipe found on website.

Fueling The Body Properly

In order to prevent cravings of bad foods and starches one needs to know what the body requires. God gave us the foods to properly nourish the body and prevent diseases as well as maintain an ideal weight.

Physical weakness is a demand for fuel. Those who fuel up with quick digesting sugars and starches will require fuel again soon. Those who consume foods containing large percentages of slow digesting essential fats, instead of sugar and starch, do not require energy-boosting snacks and can control their weight easily.

Our human tissue requires nourishment every morning with slow digesting proteins, omega fats and raw, long fiber foods – not starch, sugar or processed foods. If you eat mostly essential nutrients each morning you will have all day to use up any possible excess and will be able to control weight easily.

Our digestive systems function best with RAW, unprocessed foods that slowly release nutrients.

Hunger is a signal that the body requires protein. If you eat fruit and other foods without protein when you are really hungry, you will continue to be hungry. This goes the same as when you eat low-protein starches such as: cereals, breads or potatoes.

Therefore, it is very important to EAT breakfast every morning. Studies have proven that those who do not eat a well balanced breakfast are overweight or become overweight. Most people think that if they should skip a meal, it should be breakfast. You will also notice that most overweight people say, "Oh I don't eat very much and I never eat breakfast, and I just can't seem to get this weight off". This is the largest down fall I see in my clients. The meal you should skip would be dinner. However, I do not recommend skipping any meals. You cannot possibly have the energy or fuel to keep yourself going all day without breakfast. This is why people are so fatigued by mid-afternoon. They have no fuel to fire the metabolism. I teach my clients that if you cannot eat breakfast, then start small. The hemp hearts are a great way to at least get your protein. I am not saying go overboard with breakfast. A small handful will certainly do! Try eating a boiled egg, these are also great for protein and are quick to eat and easy to prepare. Boil some eggs a few days in advance. Eat some RAW fruits or nuts. Then make yourself a power boosting muffin. I have some great recipes for hemp-blueberry muffins. Yummy power food! Or try yogurt with your hemp sprinkled on it. Try to eat a whole food, not a boxed pop tart or donut. Also try to eat as much raw vegetation as you can. Try sprouts for morning, banana, or kiwi or pineapple. I believe eating a diet containing 85% raw foods will better help you live a longer, healthier and happier life. I offer you these other suggestions as I know most of you reading this will probably not want to go cold turkey and eat only raw foods. You will be amazed at how much better you will feel after enjoying a healthy breakfast. Don't forget to drink your Guyaki Yerba Mate tea as your drink for breakfast. Of course you could follow that drink with some fresh squeezed organic grapefruit, orange or apple juice!

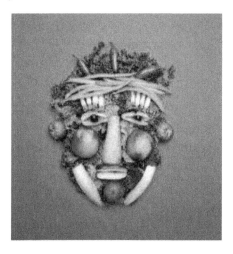

Then come mid-morning, have yourself a healthy snack such as a living whole food bar. Not to be mistaken for 'power bars' or candy bars or chips. Remember, if you must eat 'power' bars as your snack I encourage you to eat LIVING raw food bars so you get the beneficial living enzymes and pro-biotics, otherwise you are doing nothing more than satisfying your taste buds for the moment. Eat a living food bar such as Bumble Bar. RAW Revolution living bar. This is a very unique bar for all to love!

Oh the flavor and softness of it not to mention the protein and nutrient factor this wonder bar has! These are a great little bar to introduce to your kids, they love these bars! Hemp or flax seed bars or Greens food bars. These are all living raw food bars to power your cells. You can always try my recipe for raw power bites as well to satisfy your cravings! These are easy to take along to work and yummy to eat. Cacao Goji Super Food Power Snack Grab a bite of energy and celebrate, because while your taste buds are singing, your body's feeling even healthier. You can also snack on carrots, celery or an apple. During this time is a great time to incorporate your PHresh greens into your daily routine.

My favorite snack is a hand full of fresh sprouts in the 2nd day of sprouting. Sprouts contain lots of chlorophyll which helps purify the colon. Sprouts also contain protein in the purest form. Sprouts are the most reliable year-round source of vitamin C, beta-carotene, and many B vitamins (such as folacin). Sprouted Mung Beans have the carbohydrate content of a melon, vitamin A of a lemon, thiamin of an avocado, riboflavin of a dry apple, niacin of a banana, and ascorbic acid of a loganberry. Other studies have shown sprouts to be a powerful antioxidant and may assist in preventing some types of cancer. Sprouting is very economical and easy to do. You can sprout mung beans, adzuki, lentils, broccoli, alfalfa and many other legumes and beans and even rice! Sprouting is fun, easy and oh so tasteful! Check out www.seedtimetoharvest.com

for great tips on sprouting and what to do with them.

Concentrate on drinking your room temperature water or hot tea during the day as well. For optimum health benefits, I recommend drinking 5 cups of organic loose leaf herbal teas per day. Staying hydrated is essential.

Next, you are ready for lunch. This is the time for your 2nd helping of hemp hearts. Put them on salads, fish or eggs. Or eat them plain again. If you must eat out during work, don't forget to take your Yogi detox tea to rid your body of some toxins you will consume.

Mid-afternoon is another great time for one of those healthy living snack bars. You can even enjoy an energizing smoothie during this time or for mid-morning. Power smoothies are an excellent way to cleanse your body and energize as well. The smoothies I am talking about are the ones you make yourself, not the ones you go buy at smoothie shops that may have all sorts of MSG's or sugars in them. This is also a great time for that 2nd glass of ACV mixture. Eating fruit at this time is also a good idea. Grapes are the fruit of choice or blueberries

Power Smoothie

1 & 1/2 Cup Almond or Hemp Bliss or even RAW real milk

1 banana

½ Cup blueberries

3 Tablespoons Hemp Seeds

2 Tbl. Selina Naturally Coconut Oil

1 scoop Manitoba Harvest (Pro Fiber)

2 Tbl. Navitas Naturals Raw Cocoa Powder

1 Tbl. PHresh Greens

Mix in blender, do NOT add ice. If you need it thinner, add more milk. Then drink up and enjoy!

You can find tons of other healthy recipes on my website and in my good friend, Liana Werner-Gray's book, The Earth Diet. *www.theearthdiet.com*

When you get home after work it's dinner time. Have yourself a healthy balanced meal trying to avoid pork at all cost. Red meat is fine and so is chicken and fish if you are a meat eater, keeping in mind to only buy meat that has been certified organic and or kosher in a local health food store. Also, please try to limit your meat intake to 1 time per week. We do not need meat for every meal of the day or ever every week. If you buy the mass produced meat at chain grocery stores, then you are defeating the purpose of purifying your body as these meats are tainted with hormones and poisons. It is best to find a local farmer whom raises their own meat cattle or bison. Bison is so much lower in fat and a very good meat for you. Better yet, find and harvest your own meat or seek out a farmer near you. Just ask your local health food stores where the meat farmers are hiding. Again, I cannot stress the importance of eating humanely raised and harvested meats. Eating RAW as much as possible will give your body optimum health and wellness.

I personally do not eat chicken or turkey or any fowl. I have been vegetarian for years, but in August of 2011, my holistic kidney doctor turned me in to a part time carnivore. I am to eat red meat that is raised on a natural grass fed diet and organic farms. Ask me more about this in email. I am semi vegetarian as I only eat wild caught salmon and fresh sushi, but not bottom dweller sushi and I try to do raw foods as much as possible. As mentioned, I practice the 80/20 rule, meaning I eat 80% RAW and 20% cooked or heated to 118 degrees. I do not insist on everyone becoming vegetarian, semi-vegetarian or vegan. Each person has his/her own needs. However, I do not encourage anyone being totally vegan as it is very hard to get your amino acids and nutrients this way. (of course hemp is the alternative) Although, I do have some fantastic Vegan friends in which this life style works well for them. As you will get to know me, I believe in 'Balance'. I believe that NOT every human is the same and not every one of us can eat just alike. Also keep in mind that if you have been in a toxic world and have fallen ill or allergic to certain foods, then there are certain measures and foods you need to adjust. We have to find out what got us to the point of sickness and how we need to remedy that sickness. Once we have purged our body of all toxins, and bad foods and poisons from the environment, then we can start incorporating the foods we have loved...but the foods we loved will of course need to be 100% Organic. It has also been proven that vegans are at a high risk of brain tumors, this especially increases if you eat tofu.

Remember to always to try to eat your dinner by 6 or 7 p.m. as this gives the body ample time to digest all the food it has taken in. If you can go for a short walk right after dinner, that is great. Walking gives the body something to do with those fats it just processed. Then if you must have a snack before bed, try to snack by 8 p.m. Make that snack an organic semi-tart apple or half of an avocado with cracked pepper. This allows the body to absorb the other nutrients it has and also helps you to not be starving when you wake up in the morning. I always have my snack before bed. As usual, I alternate what snack I eat each evening.

Eat as many colors of the rainbow as you can. The more colorful the food are the better. I know you have heard this time and again, but it's stands to be true. Try to eat as much organic as possible. This way you are assured to get the appropriate vitamins and minerals. This has been the ancient rule of thumb and still holds true today.

I also suggest you add a fresh salsa to your daily diet. Or at least incorporate it as much as possible. Try to stick with medium or hot. Salsa has so many essential vitamins and minerals. (tomatoes, red and green peppers, garlic, onions jalapenos and red wine vinegar) Also salsa is great for the boost of metabolism and getting your heart rate going. As salsa tends to be spicy or hot, this gets the adrenals going, therefore allowing your body to faster convert the fat to energy. The hotter the better! Salsa is great on eggs, omelets, bean burritos or rice. You can put salsa on almost anything. Eating fresh guacamole is also as important for the beneficial fat found in this amazing fruit.

*Also a helpful tip: When eating, always chew slowly, this allows the vitamins and enzymes to be better absorbed into your body for better digestion. This is something to consider, when you do not properly absorb and digest your nutrients, it throws your body off and you get stuck in your rut. You may be eating all the greatest of foods, but if your body is not absorbing the nutrients or properly digesting them, you are eating in vain. You may want to consider getting some good digestive enzymes and check with your natural practicing doctor to have you tested to see how well you are absorbing your nutrients. This can be due to not having a proper cleansing routine and getting all the toxins out of your body. As mentioned earlier, it is very important to do a full body cleanse at least once per year. Some people require two times per year until they have achieved their mission of eliminating toxins. If you chew your food very slowly, this helps you to pull away from the table. Speaking of table, I highly suggest that you eat your meals sitting at the dinner table NOT in front of the TV. Why? Well sitting at the table, you are more likely to sit up straighter and this aids in digestion as well. When you are sitting on the couch in front of the TV all snug, then you have poor posture and you tend to eat more because you are comfortable and engaged in the TV program. Just an observation: not everyone who sits in front of the TV and eats is overweight, but good chances are that everyone who is overweight sits in front of the TV while eating. TV is not a good thing to have in your home anyway...to much bad stuff on there and too many 'Big Pharma' lies being poisoned in people's brains.

When you are snacking on raw healthy snacks, then standing up is perfect! For instance, walking through the mall, through the office or doing house chores are great times to snack on healthy foods.

As you can see, I promote eating and then eating again! When eating proper portions, you will not be as hungry and your body can absorb your food intake much quicker and convert it to energy. Not to be confused with 'Live to Eat' mentality. We should "Eat to Live'! Also, keep in mind, your body did not get in the condition it is in over-night, so it will not get in great health over night as well. You are retraining your brain and re-booting your system. So slow down and enjoy and savor the new transformations.

So now you are probably thinking that if the previous mentioned staples are supposed to curb my appetite – then why am I being told to eat more times per day?   Well that's the beauty of this regimen – you get to enjoy food! You do not deprive yourself, ever. You may find that you just do not have a craving at all to eat anything since you have incorporated these staples in your diet.   However, you still need to *fuel* your body with good enzymes. You can get all enzymes you need from food. However, if you are just now making the change from mainstream food to pure wholesome 'REAL' food, then it could be possible that your body may not be absorbing the vitamins you are consuming. Therefore I would recommend visiting your health care provider and finding out if you are properly absorbing them.   Chances are very high that you are not absorbing nutrients. If not, then a good digestive enzyme may be appropriate for you.

There is a great company called, Core Health Products.   www.corehealthproducts.com   Core Health was founded by Shan Stratton who is known as the "Nutritionist to the Pro's" and has worked with professional sports teams such as the New York Yankees, Boston Red Sox and a host of other athletes and teams from MLB, NFL, NBA, NHL, WNBA, PGA, Collegiate and Olympic teams. His company has formulated some awesome digestive enzymes that help your body break down and utilize the nutrients from your cooked foods along with eliminating the toxins your body cannot handle. Core Health's motto is *Nutrient utilization is more important than just nutrient consumption.*

Yes, even me, your Organic Guru, takes digestive enzymes. Remember we discussed earlier about all the toxic sludge we carry in our colon. This is due to the constant depletion of our soils and the over sprays from non-organic farms. Therefore, even the cleanest of diets such as mine, still need that extra shove to get those harmful toxins OUT and start ABSORBING more nutrients. This is why I love Core Health Products, due to the nature of their formulation. They have other products as well to help give you that extra boost we all need from time to time and without any synthetic ingredients.

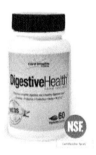

Why Do My Supplements Need To Be Organic?

A supplement is a supplement is a supplement right? No not at all. Sure the FDA and supplement making companies can label them as supplements, but how much are they really 'supplementing' your body? What kind of nutrients are really in these so called supplements? How are they made? Just like the sources of your food supply in which you need to know where it comes from and what was used to grow the foods, the same holds true to your vitamins/supplements. It is very important to know the source of the supplement and how they are made. If you are taking supplements with added fillers such as non-organic ingredients and fillers and preservatives then it is just like eating that apple with pesticides sprayed on it. These additives deplete the nutritional value of the supplement. Why even take the supplements if they are not real sources from organic herbs and plants? You should not, period! It is often a puzzle to people's minds that when they become sick, ill or diseased they always say, "Oh my, how could this happen, I take all my recommended vitamins and supplements and I eat my veggies". The answer is again, simple yet broad. You see, if you are consuming products that are artificial and have little nutritional value, then ask yourself, how in the world can this be healthy or beneficial for you? Of course the ideal means of taking care of our bodies would be simply through our food supply and only depend on the foods we consume to take care of our missing nutrients and vitamins. This is the ideal world and the ideal world of our ancestors. However, even with the most clean and toxic free eaters, myself included, we still get that 4 – 8% over spray of the pesticides, chemtrails and infected soils to run over into our plates. This causes us not to be able to properly 'absorb' our vital nutrients. Therefore, in this day and time even our 100% organic food supply has been tainted by the air pollution, the water pollution and the toxic soils. Therefore, we must supplement our bodies with the needed vitamins and enzymes we were meant to have to maintain optimum health. The truth of the matter is that most OTC supplements and even most of those found in your organic health food stores are NOT organic and have unnecessary fillers and binders for the gel caps, plus they have very little of the actual vitamin that is being advertised in the pill. Also if you are taking that supplement that has additives and preservatives, then you might as well be just taking a tic tac that touts vitamin c. Like my friend Shan Stratton of Core Health Products says, taking Vitamin C as ascorbic acid is only one part of the whole food form so we should always strive for whole food sources in all of our supplementation.

I hope you are following me here. You see it is very necessary that we FUEL our bodies with the proper nutrition and as clean of nutrients as we possibly can. Although some diseases and ailments may sneak into our own lives, there is always a way to reverse those ailments. We cannot possibly think that if we continue consuming those fake capsules and fake supplements we will continue to have the most vibrant health. It just does not work that way, for instance if you fill your gas tank with gas and you put the proper oil in the system, then your car is always going to run smoothly and have a very long life if you nurture it. However, if you start adding a little water with that gas, and get an oil mixed with water, salt or whatever, sure your car will still run for a while, but then after a while of continually absorbing all those foreign fillers, the car begins to wear down and eventually shut down. This is how our bodies work, our liver and kidneys cannot continue on a long road of fake nutrients and vitamins. Know your sources of any vitamin, supplement or even holistic pain reliever. As always, the better you take care of your body, the better your body takes care of you!

FAT, that's where it's At!

If you are continually fueling your body with healthy fat burning foods, then there will be no need to watch your calorie intake. I have been eating this way for years and I cannot tell you the last time I got concerned about how many calories were in something I ate. To be honest with you, my fat gram and calorie intake is off the charts. I do consume over 2000 calories per day and my fat consumption is well over 100 grams. I do not say this to brag or gloat but to inform you of the power of food. I could have never eaten this way with the mainstream food industry's 'faux' stuff they call food! I am also NOT telling you to go out and consume thousands of calories or hundreds of fat grams per day.

Again, when you eat the proper fats and calories without gorging yourself, and when you eat CLEAN chemical free foods then they will work for the betterment of your health. It's all about *'fueling'* your brain.

As I mentioned at the beginning of this book, calorie, fat and point counting is NOT important. Rather, the kind and quality of food is important. With my guidance through consultations, you will begin to understand what the benefits of food really are. You will understand the value of food. You will view food in a completely different light. Why not make food work FOR you instead of against you?

Good Facts About Fat

Fat supplies your body with essential fatty acids. These are acids that your body needs in order to function properly, but doesn't make on it's own. Since your body can't make them, it must get these essential fatty acids from food sources.

Fat carries fat-soluble vitamins around the body. Vitamins A, D, E, and K are brought into the body transported around to where they are needed by fat. Fat helps maintain healthy skin. In children, fat helps promote proper eyesight and brain development.

Of course, all fat isn't good. There are negative aspects to fat as well, which is why you've been warned for so long about a high fat diet. People have been eating the wrong fats, reading the wrong labels and listening to the wrong media outlets about fats.

Bad Facts About Fat

Myth: Fat has twice as many calories as carbohydrate and protein.

Myth: Fat can increase your risk for heart disease or stroke.
Myth: Some fats can raise blood cholesterol. High

cholesterol contributes to clogged arteries and deprives the heart and brain of vital oxygen-rich blood.

It's important to figure out how to derive the benefits of good fats while avoiding the risks associated with bad fats. This means learning more about "good" fats and "bad" fats and finding out how much fat you should personally have in your daily diet. Taking fat completely out of one's diet in order to lose weight is a step backwards and can create a myriad of preventable health problems, especially when good fat can assist with weight loss. I know this because that is exactly what I did for 2 years of my life! Goodness, I was a health nut I thought. Hey, if my fat intake only totaled to 25 grams per day I was a health machine, so I thought! Funny, I would read the label all right, but only the part where it told me the amount of fat grams. Oh yay, this oatmeal pie only has 8 fat grams therefore I have 17 more grams till I hit my limit! Oh boy, now I can go snack on those trail mixes and "baked" chips to avoid over consuming of fat grams. Then I would eat lots and lots of pasta as this only accounted for about 3% of my fat intake. Oh boy I was on the right track now! I can eat what I want as long as I don't exceed the 'fat' intake.

Somehow, it just never clicked WHY in the world I had continual gas pains, constipation and very low blood pressure. My body must be just stupid I thought, because after all I am the "health queen"! Oh geeze, if I only knew then. As I mention to all of you, where there is life there IS hope. I obtained many ailments throughout my 2 year reign with the 'low fat' crown. After I was awakened to the facts of the actual good fats and how our body's need these beneficial medium chain fatty acids, I was on my road to recovery and reversing all my complaints, even over coming all my kidney ailments in which I acquired after my surgery of the ripe young age of 8. After my surgery, I suffered many problems with my kidneys for 25 years! I was sent to the emergency room and hospitalized for a day year after year. Sometimes they would send me home with 106 degree temperature insisting I had the flu! Then I would have to go back due to so much pain. Finally they would believe that I actually had kidney surgery. Then the docs would put me on a kidney flush and send me home with Rx water pills and infection miracle pills. Enough was enough.

After our son's episodes of 27 surgeries we were introduced to an alternative practicing doctor in Denver, CO. This doctor enlightened us on the facts of foods and the fact that you really are what you eat, more importantly, you are what you digest and your children are what the mother digest. With that being said, I was on my life's mission to get healthy and stay out of the hospitals and have my son disease free. This is exactly what I did, therefore passing my research of foods and facts along to you. So you see, my friends, you can do this too. This can benefit all your health concerns. You just first must be re-programmed if you will. I mean this in the kindest way. I too had to be 're-programmed'. I am so thankful to my friends, classes and books I had access to. I would not have been able to bring you enlightenment if I had not gone through these horrible trials myself. Not that I suggest you make it bad before it gets good, but rather I bring to you my own insights by my own mistakes and my own ailments, diseases and pains. So please ponder on the facts I state throughout this short book. Remember our trusted friend Organic Extra Virgin Coconut Oil?

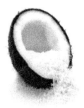

Let me remind you of why this is so good for our health. Although remember you have been misguided by the media and food industry by having you believe this oil is detrimental to one's health. Just think about it, we need some fats to nourish our bodies, we need some of those good fats to combat the bad fats and to fuel our cells to protect us from the harmful bacteria which causes infections that lead to diseases.

Let's take a look.

Myth: Saturated Fats present in Coconut Oil adds to body weight and leads to obesity.

Fact: On the contrary, the Medium Chain Fatty Acids (Saturated Fats) present in Coconut Oil increases rate of metabolism thereby leading to higher consumption of energy for metabolic activities and resultant burning of more fats. In fact, coconut oil is prescribed for losing weight and a systematic intake of coconut oil will help you lose a considerable amount of weight.

Myth: Coconut Oil is sweet to taste and not good for diabetics.

Fact: This oil tastes like any other oil and is not sweet (How it can be when it has only fats and no glucose in it!). Moreover, this oil promotes secretion of insulin from pancreas and thus helps control diabetes. Recent experiments have proved that regular uses of coconut oil can greatly reduce the chances of diabetes.

Myth: This oil is thick and is not absorbed easily.

Fact: Coconut oil, and more so the Virgin Coconut Oil, is thin, non-sticky and non-greasy and is readily absorbed. That is why coconut oil is preferred for massaging and as tanning oil. Remember earlier I stated the fact is that this is both Anti-fungal and Anti-bacterial. Great for skin irritations and believe it or not...ACNE! Yes, this helps to actually clear acne infections. My daughter did not believe this at all and refused to put this on her skin because of the high oil content. Then when she finally broke down and just tried it at night time only, wow, did she see the improvement. Of course she would not let me know I was right, she would just ask me where the coconut was each night.

*Some of these facts and myths were taken from the www.organic.net website. *Other inserts taken from www.coconut-oil-central.com

The nutritional facts on organic unrefined coconut oil is impressive! They're so good that deceitful authorities in connivance with coconut oil's competition intentionally buried them away from your knowledge.

Before the 1930s, Americans used coconut oil *a lot* in their food preparation and heart disease was virtually unheard of. After the tropical oils war, coconut oil finally succumbed to a barrage of disinformation campaigns and *hydrogenated* vegetable oils, mainly from soybeans, won out.

It didn't take long for many Americans to develop and suffer from *heart disease* at an alarming rate. And decades later, *obesity* is now an epidemic in the US.

Because of you know what, they replaced a completely beneficial *saturated* oil that has been used for ages with *unsaturated* ones that are composed of toxic *trans fatty acids*.

The Big Difference

Most other oils or fats are *long-chain fatty acids (LCFA)* by enlarge. Coconut oil contains predominantly *medium-chain fatty acids (MCFA)* and *no* trans-fats.

MCFAs are what truly defines this amazing tropical oil. Many experts conveniently treat the terms MCFAs and coconut oil as synonyms. And as you'll see, MCFA-rich coconut oil is so much different from LCFA-oils such as soybean oil.

MCFAs are an excellent source of fuel *to power your metabolism.* Upon entering the intestinal tract, they are quickly absorbed into the portal vein and sent straight to your liver to create energy.

LCFAs, on the other hand, have to circulate your bloodstream. If you have a low thyroid function *(hypothyroidism)* especially, a few of these molecules is enough to create even more body fat to be stored away as love handles, for one.

What about Avocados? Well let's just see about these beauties. Oh so many benefits from this God given fruit! Yes, they are a fruit and not a vegetable.

The Aztec word for avocado was *ahuacatl,* which means "testicle tree".

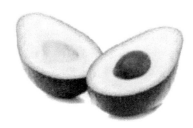

Spanish explorers could not pronounce *ahuacatl,* so they called the avocado origin of guacamole is the Aztec avocado sauce called *ahuaca-hulli.* The average avocado contains 300 calories and 30 grams of healthy polyunsaturated and monounsaturated fat. Avocados have the highest protein content of any fruit. Avocados contain more potassium than bananas. One avocado contains 81 mcg of <u>lutein</u>, an important nutrient for healthy eyes. I could eat guacamole every day, and I do just about! aguacate. This is the origin of the word guacamole.

Avocados, due to their mono and polyunsaturated fat content, are a great substitution for foods rich in saturated fat. Avocados also contribute nearly 20 vitamins, minerals and beneficial plant compounds that can contribute to the nutrient quality of your diet. Avocados are very low in Cholesterol and Sodium. They are also a good source of Dietary Fiber, Vitamin E (Alpha Tocopherol) and Copper, and a very good source of Vitamin C.

Health Benefits

Avocado is a fruit that is often avoided because of its high fat content. Together with that perception, the numerous health benefits are also overlooked. It's time we take a good look at the healing virtues of this fruit:

Bad breath: The avocado is one of the best natural mouth wash and a remedy for bad breath. It is effective in removing intestinal putrefactions or decomposition which are the real cause of a coated tongue and this unpleasant condition.

Beauty aid: The oil extracted is widely used in preparation of beauty products. These include creams, cleansers and moisturizers to prevent the ageing effect of dehydration; bath oils, shampoos, scalp conditioner and hair tonic. Also a great mask for use two to three times per week. Just simply mash a very ripe avocado then apply to face and neck, leave on for 30 minutes then rinse. This harden to a clay like mask and when rinsed off, makes your skin feel like a baby's bottom. Ahhh, the joys of home remedies and very inexpensive alternatives to those costly face creams in a jar. Just go "pick" (yes pun intended) your own mask! Then follow up with some awesome avocado oil that you can get at your local grocer or health food store. Straight, pure avocado oil, yes the kind you cook or make salad dressings with! Just do not get the kind with herbs infused in it. For a some great home recipes to pamper yourself with, study my skin chapter in here.

Blood pressure: The high potassium and folate content in avocado helps to regulate blood pressure, protecting your body against circulatory diseases, heart problems and stroke.

Cholesterol: An avocado contains oleic and linoleic acids that are effective in lowering the LDL cholesterol and increasing the healthy HDL cholesterol.

Eyesight: The potent anti-oxidant content in avocado helps neutralize free radicals that are important for improving eyesight and prevent eye problems like astigmatism, cataracts and glaucoma.

Fetal development: The high folate content is important and necessary for healthy fetal cell and tissue development.

Immune system: Regular consumption of avocados strengthens the body's immune system.

Increases absorption of phytonutrients: Studies have proven that when even a small amount of avocado is consumed together with other fruits and vegetables, the absorption of phytonutrients are a few times higher than when consumed on its own. This alone makes it worthwhile to be eating avocados regularly.

Kidney stones: Consumption of the high-potassium content fruit helps to reduce urinary calcium excretion, lowering the risk of stones forming in the kidney.

Muscle and nerve: The high potassium content helps balance our body's electrolytes, aids muscle activity, nerve function and energy metabolism.

Prostate cancer: Studies have shown that certain unique phytonutrient substances in avocados have been known to help prevent the growth of prostate cancer cells and may even help repair the damaged cells.

I could go on and on about other good fatty foods, but there are so many to give to you. I just wanted to give you the two most high fat foods that the media wants you to steer clear of. So now you will have the knowledge to research the type of fat your oil has.

Keep in mind, food is NOT rocket science! We should be able to enjoy foods and not worry about what is in what and medium chain fatty acids or omega's 3, 6 and 9's. Now these are very important points of fat and why they work, but if we eat what our Creator intended and what He gave us in the pure form, then we should not worry how many, what kinds or which ones and what time. We will have the common sense to eat pure wholesome 'Fuel for our Body' kind of food. I mean it's no wonder with all the "you can't eat this, you can't eat that' information out there that our nation is very confused on food matters. First, this food is great for you, next thing you know, it will kill you!

It's really easy. Just avoid chemical infested foods and bleached and chlorinated foods like the plague and you will see your ailments reverse and your health burst with energy and your biological age actually reverse! Let's go back to the basics with our food and way of life. Stop the GMO's, the chemicals and all the preservatives in the foods.

What are GMOs?

GMOs (or "genetically modified organisms") are organisms that have been created through the gene-splicing techniques of biotechnology (also called genetic engineering, or GE). This relatively new science allows DNA from one species to be injected into another species in a laboratory, creating combinations of plant, animal, bacteria, and viral genes that do not occur in nature or through traditional crossbreeding methods.

Are GMOs safe?

In 30 other countries around the world, including Australia, Japan, and all of the countries in the European Union, there are significant restrictions or outright bans on the production of GMOs, because they are not considered proven safe. In the U.S. on the other hand, the FDA approved commercial production of GMOs based on studies conducted by the companies who created them and profit from their sale. Many health-conscious shoppers find the lack of rigorous, independent, scientific examination on the impact of consuming GM foods to be cause for concern.

*Excerpts taken from the Non-GMO Project
www.nongmoproject.org

I don't know about you, but if there is the slightest chance of the gmo being harmful, I don't want to take the chance. Also if other countries are banning such practices, then wouldn't you wonder why? Why take the chance when you can have gmo free foods? Remember, I grew up on these Monsanto farms which was the culprit to my kidney failure and surgery at the age of 8. Then my son was born with a deadly disease that was related to not just GMO, but all the toxins in my body from round –up, pesticides and herbicides. Not to mention all the MSG (mono-sodium glutamate). However, just REMEMBER that because a food is NON GMO does NOT in any way mean that it is FREE from chemicals such as round-up, pesticides or herbicides. Inquire within for my seminars on this controversial topic. The key words we want for our food supply is TOXIC FREE! This will assure us of any harmful ingredients getting in our food supply. Take a peek at our website www.pureintegrityverified.com to find out about our PURE INTEGRITY VERIFIED™ Seal of Approval. This IS the seal to be on the look-out for in 2014 and 2015. This seal stamps the strict approval on the company as a WHOLE. We qualify the entire company, not just one single product. As we believe in a toxic free planet. We believe in Pure Integrity,

Trust and future generations' health. Together, we will make a difference in the health of our nation.

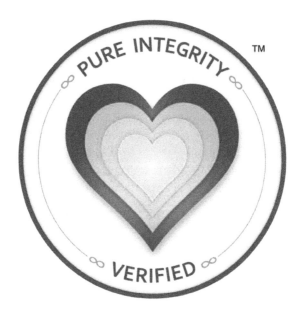

What is MSG? Monosodium Glutamate

MSG is a product produced from fruits vegetables, grains, fish, meat, poultry, and/or bacteria. When used in pharmaceuticals it is called a pharmaceutical. When used in food, it is called a food. Often, but not always, MSG is used in processed food as a flavor enhancer.

Simply stated, MSG is glutamic acid that has been manufactured in a food or chemical plant or created by fermentation. In every case, the glutamic acid that has been manufactured in food or chemical plants or created by fermentation is accompanied by unwanted byproducts of manufacture referred to as impurities.
Unprocessed/unadulterated/unfermented protein in any meat, fish, fruit, grain, vegetable etc., contains glutamic   acid   but   no   impurities.
Unprocessed/unadulterated/unfermented
mushrooms and tomatoes contain glutamic acid, but they do not contain MSG.

Prior to 1957, MSG was made by extracting glutamic acid from protein. Some MSG is still made that way, but since 1957, MSG has also been produced using genetically modified bacteria (genetically modified organisms or GMO's), that secrete glutamic acid through their cell walls. MSG can be extracted from any food that contains protein. Similarly, when any protein is fermented, MSG (glutamic acid that has been released from protein by the fermentation process) will be formed.

The key to understanding MSG lies in understanding the fact that MSG is a product (something manufactured or processed), not a substance found in nature without adulteration (changing) it.

Regardless of the way in which it was produced, MSG contains unwanted substances referred to as impurities. MSG causes adverse reactions in people who ingest amounts that exceed their tolerances for the substance.   Unadulterated, unprocessed, unfermented protein, which contains glutamic acid, does not cause adverse reactions.

Ingredients that contain MSG can be added to processed foods, or MSG can be formed or created during processing.

For more detailed information about this silent killer, please refer to www.fuelforthebody.org and check out the MSG tab.

Be Careful What You MEAT!

11

Most Americans give little or no thought to the origin of the 'food' they are consuming. Many think food is 'safe' because it is regulated by the USDA and the FDA. Yet as the continuation of the e-coli infections show, this is not the case. You will be surprised of what the USDA and FDA turns their heads on. Again, I will discuss this in my 2nd book about what the evil empire has been hiding from us all these years.

Since 2003, food borne illness continues to sicken an estimated 76 million, hospitalize 325,000 and kill 5,000 Americans each year! (taken from www.law.msu.edu/king) Poor sanitation causes these pathogens to contaminate meat during sloppy high-speed slaughter. There are machines in slaughter houses that rip out the intestines of animals, spilling fecal matter containing e-coli and other pathogens onto meat intended for consumption. The USDA now considers feces a 'cosmetic blemish' allowing workers to rinse it off and further process it for consumption. Also fear and pain cause animals to produce hormones which damage their meat and are toxic. This is what you eat my friends!

Animals in slaughter houses can see, smell and hear the slaughter of those before them. I do not want to go into gory details here. I will however recommend checking out: www.law.msu.edu/king and www.all-creatures.org . Also some great documentaries are Food Inc., Dirt, Food Matters and Fast Food Nation. Keep in mind that I believe some of the animal activist have taken some things a bit too far.

Animals are God's creatures. Yes He put some animals on this planet for the human food chain. However, the means that are used in our modern world today was not what our Creator had in mind. Just because I am semi-vegetarian and I stand up for animal rights, does NOT mean I protest "humane" hunters or "humane" killing of the farm animals for food. Humane is the key word here. If you shoot an animal (for food of course) in the wild then they have no idea their death was coming and are dead before they knew what happened. They have no time to get scared or have fear rushing through them to intoxicate the meat. I believe this is how God intended animals to be harvested. Yes God gave us the 'divine right' to have 'dominion' over animals. That does NOT give us the right to torture and abuse an animal. There are many organic farmers near you in which butcher their own cattle, bison or lamb. They raise happy, healthy animals and are humanely put down without fear or torture. So you see, I am NOT against raising animals for food – I am against the disgusting and horrific ways the food industry tries to make the mighty dollar at the animal's expense. Also keep in mind that it is extremely important to raise animals on their natural diets. For instance, cows, bison, deer and elk are NOT corn, soy or meat eaters. They eat the grasses and foliage of the earth. If the animal is not fed it's natural diet, then that animal cannot produce the proper L-carnitine. The animal needs this L-carnitine to function properly.

L Carnitine is not an amino acid, but a substance related to the B vitamins. However, due to its chemical structure, which is similar to those amazing amino acids it is usually considered together with them.   It's primary role is to help transport fatty acids into the energy producing units in the cells - the mitochondria, where they can be converted to energy. This is a major source of energy for the muscles, including those of the heart. As such, carnitine increases the use of fat as an energy source.

Carnitine is manufactured by the body if sufficient amounts of iron, vitamin B_1, vitamin C, niacin, vitamin B6, lysine, and methionine are available. Carnitine also enhances the effectiveness of antioxidant vitamins C and E.

Carnitine is often referred to as a protein-like substance or a vitamin-like substance.

A carnitine derivative – an ester called acetyl-l-carnitine is thought to slow the aging of the brain as well as other nerve cells.   Keep in mind that the animal MUST be fed an all natural diet. Meaning the animal must eat what it was intended to eat, such as a cow is NOT a meat eater, nor is it a grain animal. They are GRASS eaters. The cow cannot produce it's own carnitine if it is fed an unnatural diet, or even if it is fed half grass and half grain. Find out more on this subject from my friend Trish Strawn at Growing Synergy. She has some great insight on the way an animal is to be raised, fed, harvested   and   maintained. www.growingsynergy.com

Think about it. If we knew what went on in slaughter houses, we would be way to scared to eat any meat what so ever from food industry grocery stores. I encourage you to watch the movie: Food Matters and of course Food Inc. These documentaries will definitely make you stop and think.

Same goes for the fish industry. Fish are good to eat. Personally I eat sushi or seared salmon & tuna. Being careful where I eat my sushi as not to get tainted fish. I go to Japanese restaurants and get to know the chef and owners. This way you can ask questions and know where the meat comes from. It is best to eat only fish that have BOTH fins and scales. This helps reduce the mercury and pollution intake the fish would have and these fish would not be bottom feeders. Bottom feeders, yuck! I used to eat those bottom dwellers until I really looked into their diet. Eew, they eat remains and feces on the bottom of the ocean! They are considered the cock roaches of the sea. When I stopped eating them, I ate some several months later and felt very nauseated. So there is something to be said about bottom dwellers.

Most people like to think it would be best to only buy farm raised to avoid mercury. Well this would be a good idea, however fish are raised just like cattle. Have you seen fish hatcheries? They are way over crowded in 1 barrel eliminating all the feces in the same barrel. Ugh, yuck! So now what happens? Well the fish farmers put tons of chemicals to keep the water clear so it does not look contaminated. They are also fed hormones and other un-natural substances to make them grow faster and produce

In Leviticus 11, God points out which animals He designed to be eaten. The Bible calls these animals "clean."

rapidly. So now you are eating chemical infested poop! I think I'll take my chances on the wild blue ocean and pick up less contamination of feces and chemicals. At least the ocean is free flowing constantly cleansing itself of pollution. Yes, there is a mercury problem, this is why it is important to eat fish with only both fins and scales. I will go into further detail in my 3rd book entitled: 'What Does Our Creator Have to Say About Our Food & Health'? This book will be geared to my Christian friends who call me "radical" and said God made everything clean.

Well with that standard, then I suppose eating a vulture or a rat would be just fine and dandy! There is a reason God told us not to eat certain creatures. Some creatures He put for our food chain, some creatures He put here for the circle of life! Here's just a glimpse of what the Bible says about eating the creatures of the waters.

For example, clean mammals have a "split hoof" and "chew the cud." These include cows, sheep and goats. Pigs have a split hoof but do not chew the cud and pigs do not have sweat glands to excrete the toxins in their bodies; therefore pork was not designed to be food by God's standards.

Fish that have fins and scales were designed to be food. These fish include salmon, snapper and tuna. Catfish, on the other hand, have fins but no scales, and they dwell on the bottom and scavenge for food....eeew! So they are considered unclean and not designed for food. Same goes for shellfish such as lobster, oysters and shrimp, they don't have fins or scales.

Ok, I know you are all scared about the Fukushima radiation. Well, the oceans are larger than the earth. Yes, true we are destroying the planet, but we have a vast blue deep sea that can replenish and filter when man leaves it alone. There are many sick fish, there are many fish being over fished and starting to become extinct. This madness must stop. Again, know your sources of fish.

Most poultry, like chicken, turkey, duck and goose, are considered clean, since they are not listed with the unclean scavenger birds like vultures.

Again, I am not trying to 'preach' to you or to tell you what is and is not a sin. I am simply pointing out some factual information as to why certain creatures should not be eaten. God knows best for us and our health and when you look at these creatures you understand why some of them are not for the human food chain!

As I mentioned previously, I will go into full detail about the Creator's idea of a healthful, vibrant and radiant life in my 3rd book.

God has designed the human body so that it is a finely-tuned instrument that is the most resilient on earth. It can endure fractures and, constant pain and great stretches of feats.

However, it is a fragile instrument because it is not built to handle excess, whether in the form of nourishment, fuel or additives. Unlike machines, it chokes on poisons when ingested in unending doses and mistaken for fuel.

Moo-ving Along To Dairy Foods

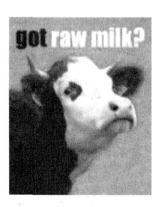

Compliments of royalty free pictures

This is a controversial subject. I recently, about 3 years ago, quit eating all dairy products to see how it would affect my health. Keeping in mind, I was only drinking the 'organic' version of pasteurized and homogenized milk products. When I stopped eating cheese or drinking milk, I found that my digestion greatly improved. I found that I did not even need or crave the milk, butter or cheese any longer. I significantly decreased my husband's intake of cheese and milk as well. He was still continuing to have some bouts with his sinus problem. Although most of his ailments with this were gone since he became diet soda free 4 years ago!!! However after studying that dairy products were a huge factor in mucus abnormalities, I realized the amount of cheese and milk he was consuming and knew it had to be what made him keep flaring up on occasion. Also keep in mind he was not consuming these products in the raw and un-pasteurized state. Just because it is 'organic' does not mean it is raw, nor does it mean it is not pasteurized. So we decreased his intake to almost NO dairy at all. Tommy thought he would just die without his 'vice' of cheese! Well he soon learned how to manage after he felt so much better. He has had no sinus infections since stopping all cheese and milk and he is no longer using nose spray. Yay! We do substitute with almond, hemp and coconut milk. These are great alternatives for granola, baking, un-baking and so on. They are delicious as well as nourishing. When we are in areas where we have access to local raw dairy farmers, then we do get that delicious real milk.

Please keep in mind that this was the consumption of PASTEURIZED milks, cheeses and butters and before we had access to organic and real 'raw' dairy farmers. This is the culprit of becoming 'lactose intolerant'. It is NOT the milk that people become allergic to or become lactose intolerant, it is the pasteurization and homogenization of the milk. These two methods actually kill all living beneficial bacteria that we need to fight infections and help aid in proper digestion. The USDA requires these methods to be used to be able to 'lawfully' sell milk products in stores. They say this makes it "safe" for consumers.

Homogenization: (Taken from any encyclopedia or dictionary) A process in which a mixture is made uniform throughout. Generally this procedure involves reducing the size of the particles of one component of the mixture and dispersing them evenly throughout the other component. Probably the most familiar example of a homogenized product is commercially sold milk. In milk that has not been homogenized the globules of fat range in diameter from approximately 1 to 20 micrometers (millionths of a meter), or 40 to 800 millionths of an inch. This allows them to separate out from the rest of the milk if it is allowed to stand. After homogenization the globules are reduced to a range of sizes clustering closely about 1 micrometer and remain stably dispersed through the milk. Homogenization is usually accomplished by pumping the milk through a small opening at high pressure. Milk that has been homogenized is better suited for shipment in paper containers but deteriorates more rapidly than un-homogenized milk.

Pasteurization: The act or process of heating a beverage or other food, such as milk or beer, to a specific temperature for a specific period of time in order to kill microorganisms that could cause disease, spoilage, or undesired fermentation.

The act or process of destroying most microorganisms in certain foods, such as fish or clam meat, by irradiating them with gamma rays or other radiation to prevent spoilage.

Babies need the mother's milk to have the proper enzymes and nutrients to grow healthy. (Although, indulging in milk or cheeses are always inspired, IF you take time to look for dairy farmers and or companies for non-gmo verified and non-chemical infested milks and cheeses). Some will say, "we are the only creatures that do not wean ourselves from milk". While that may be true, RAW milk is good for us with all the amazing living enzymes. Please take a look at the Westin A. Price for a closer look on the benefits of consuming raw milk, cheese and butter. I am just saying if you still want to have your dairy products, make it RAW un- touched by the food industry. This will not wreak havoc on our system or membranes. Tommy can now tolerate RAW milk products on limited intake. I do however bake with butter occasionally. I believe each person is different with different needs for their body. Never use margarine!

I have been fortunate enough to get my pure, whole RAW milk straight from the cow's utter! How delicious it is...yummy. I even make my own butter from the rich cream that came with my gallon jar of milk. Nothing like the togetherness of your family all taking turns shaking the cream jar to churn butter. Oh and the taste. Wow! You just can't get any better than this pure unadulterated milk product. This is the only way I would suggest you consuming any type of milk, cheese, butter or yogurt. Only in the RAW state.

Talk about some fake foods, I do not see how they can even call margarine a food family or anything. They should just call it heated nickel and bleach! Take a look below for an over view of how margarine is made. Then you can decide if you want to consume this concoction for your feeding pleasures.

How margarine and shortenings are made

• Manufacturers start with the cheapest vegetable oils, extracted at high temperatures and pressures from corn, cottonseed, soybeans, safflower seeds and canola.

• The last fraction of oil is removed with hexane, a carcinogenic solvent.

• The oils, already rancid from the extraction process, are steam cleaned. This destroys all the vitamins and antioxidants, but pesticides and solvents remain.

• The oils are mixed with a finely ground nickel catalyst.

• The oils are then put in a reactor where at high temperatures and pressures, they are flooded with hydrogen gas. The molecular structure is rearranged. What goes into the reactor is a liquid oil, what comes out is a smelly, lumpy, grey semi-solid.

• Soap-like emulsifiers are mixed in to remove all the lumps.

• The oil is steam cleaned (again) to remove the odor of chemicals.

• The oil is then bleached to get rid of the grey color.

• Synthetic vitamins and artificial flavors are mixed in.

• A natural yellow color is added to margarine...as synthetic coloring is not allowed!

• The mixture is packaged in blocks or tubs and promoted to the public as a health food.

**The above information is taken from the Weston A. Price Foundation.

More on the making of foods in future books.

There are however, some companies in the industry such as Organic Valley & Tree of Life and small farmers, who have great farming practices and can provide you with some great flavorful cheese, milk, butter and yogurt.

Mostly I use coconut oil and grape seed oils. (these are dairy free) If you do not have access to raw milk from your local farmers, then the better alternative is buying only organic milks & cheese such as Tree of Life or Organic Valley in your health food stores. Although, due to regulations of grocery stores and the good ole FDA, they must pasteurize the milk. However, they do raise their cattle humanely and harvest the milk with the best of technologies and with the least amount of stress to the animals. They also have some great RAW cheeses as well as real butter and yogurt.

The nation's best source of vitamin A

The vitamin A in butter is three times as effective as the vitamin A in fish liver oils. The natural vitamin D in butter has been found to be 100 times as effective as the common commercial form of D (viosterol). Butter, prescribed by physicians as a remedy for tuberculosis, psoriasis, xerophthalmia, dental caries, and in preventing rickets, has been promptly effective.

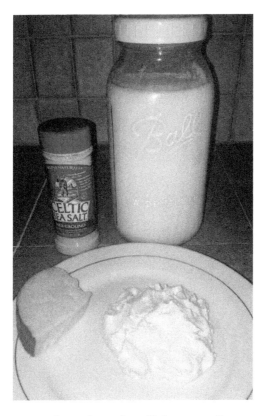

My home made real cow's milk butter.   Preserved
with salt. A block of raw cheese from my amazing
holistic farmer, Real Farm Foods of Norwood, MO.

What about produce?

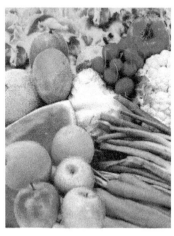

Just want to make a short observation here. You
hear all these so called 'vegetarians and or vegans'
being all radical about only eating plant based
products. Hey, no offense, I was vegetarian for
years. Recently my Holistic Kidney doctor, Dr.
Jenna Henderson, tuned me in to a part time
carnivore due to my kidney failures. (Please call or
email me for more information on this.) However,
in my observations, I notice that a lot of these
veggies/vegans are unhealthy and over-weight.
Huh? What? How can this be? I'm sure you have
seen this as well. Well for starters, did they ever
consider the 'source' of the foods they are
consuming? Did they stop to think that just because
one is vegetarian/vegan does NOT make one the

picture of health. What am I talking about? Well, the reason for the un-healthiness and over weight in certain veggies/vegans is because they simply do NOT adhere to the ORGANIC/clean food rules. They are not eating toxic free foods, not to mention they may be consuming our enemy's GMO infested veggies. This is wreaking havoc on their bodies. Sure, they have the right idea, but forgot to follow through with proper research on the source of their food supply. All I'm saying, is if you choose to be vegetarian/vegan, then be sure to make it CLEAN/ORGANIC to be as healthy as you can be.

Another point I would like to share with the over weight of these plant based eaters. They do tend to supplement their non protein intake with lots of sugars! Well this just defeats the entire purpose of being vegetarian for one's health. So please, consider your food supply before introducing it to your oral intake.

As for your produce, well these can be extremely contaminated as well. Just think of all the pesticides and fertilizers that have been sprayed all over them. All these chemicals significantly deteriorate the nutritional value of the plant. As I mentioned before, you wouldn't drink even a sip of fertilizer or pesticide so why would you eat it? Remember small quantities add up to mass quantities. Again, this is why it is important to buy organic. Look for your local farmer's markets or find a co-op in your area. These are very beneficial in keeping the consumer informed of what is going on in the food world. This will also insure to keep your local farmers in business.

Oh yes, the mass produced fruits and veggies look so appealing. My, how shiny they are! Did you ever wonder what makes them so shiny? Wax of course! Yes your pretty fruits and veggies have a wax finish on them. After all if it's pretty to the eye, then it must be good right?   Just the opposite is true. Natural and organic fruits and veggies may not be as appealing, but their nutritional value is still intact and the taste...wow, have you really tasted organic produce?   You will be amazed of the difference. When buying produce, it is best to buy all organic or locally grown. Sometimes locally grown may not be organic, however it will have less contamination as the only chemicals used on these are seven dust, some fertilizer and TLC! Sometimes, it is best to buy non local organic produce due to the harsh chemicals some farmers still use such as round-up or their trusted "miracle-grow".   You will have to ask what each farmer uses to fertilize or uses for bug repellant. Never ask, "are you organic"? Of course their answer will be "yep", as they know you are looking for organic farmers. (however some farmers are very honest and will tell you the toxins they use for their garden) You may want to also keep in mind that is does NOT matter if they are USDA certified. Some farmers may say, "well we are not 'certified', but we use no pesticides or toxic fertilizers. This is OK, as we do NOT like the USDA's biased standards. When you read my next book, you will understand more what this means.

Also locally grown is in season for the area you live in providing you with the area's best allergen defense. Let's not forget about all the genetically modifications that is happening in our veggie world. The genes are being spliced and diced as you read this.   If you only knew the truth about all the science in our foods. Don't be fooled by the FDA saying it's "OK". Remember Monsanto has its' hands, literally, in the work of the FDA. I will explain better in my next book entitled: *"Where There Is Life, There Is Hope"*.

Again, the key words are TOXIC FREE and PURE INTEGRITY VERIFIED™.   Are you beginning to catch on here?   It's all about CLEAN foods and rejecting any chemicals what so ever.   The key is NON toxic foods, REAL and natural earth foods.

It would be best to be able to grow your own organic garden. I do have my organic garden. It is delicious! Oh the joys of harvesting your first harvest. Well the joy of harvesting all your produce for that matter is self satisfying.

A   great   website   to   look   into   is, www.seedtimetoharvest.com.   Joy Scroggie offers over 35 years of organic gardening experience. She shows you how to successfully grow your organic garden in the least time possible. She also has an amazing story of how she went from almost dead to 'vibrant' and lively! She is a great raw foodist as well as a Master Gardener. I will have to add, that I do recommend eating raw as much as possible.   I practice the 80% raw and 20% cooked diet myself.

This is great to get all the living enzymes you can possibly get. It is the ultimate way to nourish and heal your body. Make it clean eating. What is your health worth to you?

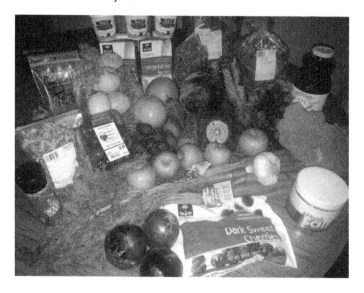

Want true health care reform? Then try investing in your kitchen pantry.

WHY ORGANIC???

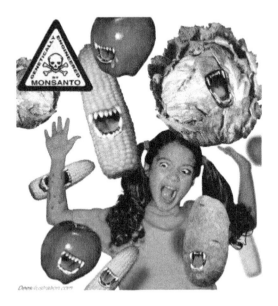

This is where the term "Frankin Foods" come from

**Photo taken from the OCA website

Well to begin with, why NOT? I get the questions often asked of me, "Why is it so important to eat organic foods? Isn't organic just another yuppy, preppy kind of life style? Isn't that what hippies and pot smokers eat? Besides, it cost so much more, why should I spend the money on the same kind of food I already eat with the organic name on it?"

All these questions have been asked. My answer is simple yet broad. To begin with, yes there is a lot of misconception of the word 'organic'. People seem to think it is just some kind of fad and hip thing that is going to "pass". They seem to think that organic is for those who are waaay out there. But that's where I do come in the picture, to shed light on these ways of thinking and put the truths on the matter and show people really what the organic world is all about. So let me start by saying, organic is NOT going to 'just pass'. Organic is indeed a word that is misused sometimes. The fact of the matter is that it is not only for yuppies, preppies and or hippies. Organic is important to us all and the well being of our soil and planet. Just because people who do smoke pot or who are true hippies does not make it wrong or crazy. We need to look at the reasoning behind the organic world. It is not a 'movement'. Organic has been around since the beginning of time, but our ancestors, grandparents called it FOOD. Organic eating & lifestyles are very important due to the fact they are pesticide, toxin and chemical free. Why do we need chemicals in our food supply? Why would you eat or drink some round up, agent orange, bug killer or miracle grow? Of course you wouldn't...but in fact you DO eat this every time you eat that food that is not clean. Now of course consuming this food is not going to kill you immediately, however it is slowly killing you and the world you live in. We were not made to absorb and digest these deadly chemicals. Just think about it. You say, but Lynnette, this is what our liver and kidneys are for, to eliminate those harmful toxins. Excuse me, but wrongo you are, our liver and kidneys are supposed to eliminate any un wanted bacteria, fungus or fillers, but not to outright rid your body of chemical pollution day after day. You say it is so expensive? Well I ask you, what is more important, your health or crap food? You are going to pay someone either by doctors or health insurance, why not pay YOUR SELF and invest in good real foods? If you look at all the sick and diseased people, you will see the foods they really do consume. Besides, have you seen the cost of cancer, insulin or heart disease lately? So think about it, you are what you eat, what do you want to be? Chemicals or a person? Never mind the fact that when you eat REAL nutrients, you actually fill your Brain instead of just filling your stomach with empty calories, therefore you actually eat more times per day , but you eat much less hence having a lower food bill as it takes less to live and be healthy on.

An organic life style is simply the act of knowing the facts. The facts are that chemical consumption wreaks havoc on your body and on the planet. So what do YOU CHOOSE? Besides the fact that non organic foods can be genetically modified, which means the food / seed has been genetically altered to create a NON natural food.

Who Says Beauty Is Only Skin Deep?

My Secrets to Glowing, Radiant & Healthy Skin

People are always asking, "How in the world is your skin always glowing and blemish free"? No I am not bragging. I just know what makes a healthy skin. As you will note below.

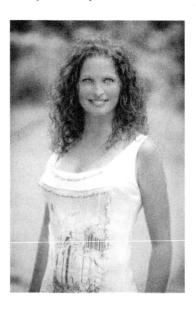

Photo by: Roxxe Photography. NO foundation, only concealer around the eyes & nose. Eyeliner, mascara & natural lip color. NO blush. Ecco Bella cosmetics. Cover photo is the same. Non-airbrushed.

FlowerColor® Makeup

As an advocate for proper skin care routines, I was ensnared by the department store skin care and make up products for years. I came from the world of cosmetics. I was the account coordinator and regional make-up artist for a large prestige make up company for over 8 years. I was the trainer to the beauty advisers' in which I held classes to teach beauty advisers' "WHY" these wonderful toxic ingredients were so good for one's skin. Yes, I taught others what I was taught. I explained the technology of the nano-capsule and the importance of it's function and how it carried the vitamin c through the product. I also explained how the lycopene in the chemicals was 'protected' and therefore giving your skin mass benefits. I could teach classes and translate formulations in my sleep.

Wow! I taught this insanity? Yes indeed I did. I was just like a mass of the public, I was UN AWARE. I was not properly educated. I was teaching what I was being taught. Well it came from the "experts" and "scientist" right? After all, these products were tested and re-tested in 7 different labs. Whew, what part of chemicals being absorbed into your blood stream did I not understand?

Just as I was enlightened, after our son's near death experiences, about foods and the food industry, I was also enlightened that OUR SKIN IS OUR LARGEST ORGAN. Wow, what a shocker that was. Duh...our skin absorbs more toxins than those being consumed orally. What goes ON your skin, goes IN your skin and in your blood stream.

Again, I went on a mission to study the other side of the make-up world. This was fairly easy, as I did not have to worry about all the 'scientific formulations'. Gee, you mean I get to put non-invasive, non-chemical based products on my skin and look great? You see, the last year of my reign as "cosmetic queen" of the department store company, my skin was actually beginning to act odd and do crazy things. How can this be? After all I was using one of the best brands on the market and all these chemicals have their purpose. Well they had their purpose all right, the purpose of your body finally rejecting these terrible toxins.

So you see, it is just a matter of time that something catches up with you. For instance, just as with eating all these chemical, GMO, MSG and artificially infested foods, the havoc they wreak will catch up with you in a matter of years. In fact, it has already caught up with people, but they just do not make the connection of fake crap and ill health or bad skin.

With all this being said, just as I mention about food....IT'S NOT ROCKET SCIENCE! Since your skin is your largest organ, then it only makes sense that if you wouldn't eat an ingredient, then do NOT put it on your skin. That is exactly what I set out to do. I gathered all food products of natural and organic of course, and experimented on my OWN skin, NO ANIMALS WERE EVER HARMED IN MY TESTING. I used all kinds of oils such as olive, grape seed, hemp oil, coconut oil and so on. I tried, making my own scrubs, cleansers and mask.

Here is what I came up with.

My daily routine varies from week to week as I like to use as much of the Earth's goodness as I can. I use an all oatmeal & sage face soap and ONLY wash ONE (1) time per day. You know the 'golden rule' of washing your face 2 and sometimes 3 times per day, like upon waking and then before bed? Geeze, what a load of caca. How does your face get dirty in bed? Um, unless you have not changed sheets in months! Even when I worked for this company, I NEVER told my clients to do this hog wash. (Unless of course you are out all day getting sweaty, muddy or playing in the ocean, then decide to go out again at night. Then of course wash when cleaning up for evening , then wash all make up off face before bed). Of course they want you to scrub, scrub, scrub, because they want to sell, sell, sell.

I will switch my face soap about every two or three weeks to an oatmeal & honey soap then to a sea kelp & red clay soap. (Keep in mind that I only use hand made or a trusted company's brand with as few ingredients as possible and sometimes I even make my own!) Then after washing, I slather my face and neck with the real deal.....our trusted medicinal plant of the Aloe Vera. Yes, your grandmother's home 'burn' remedy. This was the plant choice of Cleopatra to soak her skin in as well as her hair. Oh the wonderful cooling sensation! I let this set for a little bit while I get dressed. Aloe Vera plant is high in vitamin E and is a great 'instant face lift'. You can sleep in this and awaken with an uplifting feel and look. Of course the vitamin E does wonders for the lips. Also, by using the gel of the plant for your hair, you will see no need for hair sprays or even gels. You can adjust the amount you need depending on if you want to style your hair or just dab the ends for frizz control. It is also a great gel to massage into the scalp for dandruff remedy.

Then depending on my mood, after I have my aloe-vera already soaked in. I rub my mood oil of choice avocado, coconut or grape seed oil all over my face and neck. Ahhh, yes. (I do keep one of each of these in my kitchen and 1 of each in my vanity to not mix up with cooking) This is used as my moisturizer. Oh what an awesome glow any of these oils give your skin! I tend to use the avocado oil mostly during the day. Avocado oil is actually one of the best anti-aging solutions for your skin. Refer back to the Fat is where it's at chapter. Then I slather my entire body with the wonders of coconut oil. Radiant, simply radiant. I wait for about 5 or 10 minutes before applying any make up what so ever if I decide to wear any for the day.

I was a make-up freak in my chemical world days. These days I find that I do NOT like this stuff on my skin. So if I am in the mood for a little color, I use a little eye liner, some neutral lip liner and a neutral lip tint and if I see in the mirror that I am not satisfied with my look, then I add a concealer around my eyes and nose to even out my skin tone. If I go out at night, I will get a little dolled up by using mascara, some eye glimmers and a little color on my lips. I am not a fan of foundation at all. However, since leaving the chemical cosmetic world years ago and changing my diet and make up, I find that my skin tone has evened out and foundation is not needed. I searched for the best of the best products for my skin. The company I found that best meets my strict standards for over 6 years now is Ecco Bella. Therefore, if you do not feel you can 'make your own', then Ecco Bella is my choice for skincare. They have amazing colors as well as skin care moisturizers, eye creams and toners as well for those of you who want a 'face in a bottle'. Great news, they are all Water FREE! Of course they are FREE of anything you do not need on your skin. Free of any animal testing what so ever and free of parabens. Better yet, their packaging is made from recycled materials and use the least amount of packaging as possible. I use their Jojoba oil over my coconut oil or my avocado oil. I also use their vitamin E stick for my lip needs. Keep in mind there are a few other all natural and toxic free make up companies out there. Check into Miessence toxic free skin and body care, Giddy Organics, Akea or Devita. Again, try to make your own skin care and follow my protocols here.

At night, when I have washed my face, I apply more aloe vera plant all over my face and neck and chest. I also rub the excess in my hair. I just can't get enough of this stuff! (I use the aloe vera plant after I have done my face scrub or any mask. Please see below). Then I use my trusted coconut oil all over my face and body. (My preferred brand is Selina Naturally) I use it in my hair as a sheen for taming the frizzies during the day. It also is great for a dry scalp. In fact, coconut oil is one of my home remedies due to it's anti fungal, anti bacterial and anti-oxidant properties. Prevents pre-mature aging of skin, repairs damaged skin tissue, wards off sun damage and will help bring back youthful appearance.

Guess what teens? YOU too will reap the amazing benefits of this super oil of coconut. Did you know that this oil actually helps you to combat acne? Huh? How could it, it is so oily? Remember it is anti-fungal. This has been tried and tested positive by my daughter, Haley. (There is also true science to back this up) She did not want to admit it worked and refused to put this 'grease' on her skin for a long while. When I told her to just try it at night, well after about 5 days her face was clearing. Wow, amazing. So she secretly would come get the coconut oil from me and use it as she did not want to admit this was actually working. It helps to combat even more bacteria if you eat it. I keep one in my vanity and one in my kitchen for cooking and eating. Also, you may note that using this coconut oil all over your body on a daily basis, will help protect your skin from the harmful UVB rays.

Always keep in mind that by eating a diet RICH in anti-oxidants such as broccoli, asparagus and even eating the coconut oil (as you will note in earlier chapters) will help your body naturally protect itself from the harmful rays of the sun.

Did you know that the sun does NOT cause skin cancer? Really, you say? That's exactly right. The toxic sun screens cause skin cancer. Just look at all the ingredients in the sun screens. Remember, it is the toxins that are poisons to our body, inside and out. Although, this is a very controversial topic. Seriously, just for fun, did God create the light of the world and the humans...and say, "Haha my little earthlings, I fooled you with this amazing light in the sky. Not only do you have light to see, you have the most deadly light to human kind". Just saying. Now, I will advise you that it is possible to get sun 'poisoning'. For instance, if you are very light skinned or have not been accustomed to being in the sun for long periods of time, then it is possible to get sun poisoning if you stay in the sun and get blistered. Of course we do not want to continually burn our skin. This is why it is so important to get your DAILY intake of this lovely vitamin in the sky, called Vit. D, in small segments. Go out and enjoy your benefits once daily and let your skin drink the rays of the sun. Of course the best times to do this for the light skinned person is between the hours of noon and 4. This is when the UVB rays are the least penetrating. Remember to work your way up to longer stays in the sun. Start out with 15 minutes in sunlight if you are a very light skinned person. Also, just a tip of information for you, did you know that you need to walk out in the sunlight for 15 minutes per day with NO sunglasses on at all? Yes, your eyes need direct sunlight to enhance your vision. Vit D. to the eyes is extremely beneficial for you. More on this subject in my next book, "What Does the Creator Have to Say About our Food and Health".

Next, every other night or every 3 nights I will use my Adzuki facial scrub with my soap of choice. This is a literally crushed adzuki beans! Seems like they would really cut your skin to pieces, but actually they gently massage the skin and leave your face feeling smooth as a baby's bottom! I also want to point out that I ALWAYS use my re-usable eco-friendly BAMBOO cloth and / or silk sea sponges to wash with my face soap. These are natural exfoliators as well and very gentle on the skin for everyday use. I get my crushed Adzuki from Amber's Earth. www.ambersearth.com A great company who searched for the best of products and brings to you the wonders of this magical scrub!

Once per week I slather my face, neck and chest with HONEY while in the shower and leave on till I have washed and rinsed my hair. Oh how silky your skin is after this soak! The honey acts as a natural exfoliant for the body leaving behind the softness of the honey penetration. Honey is also great for those occasional blemishes you may encounter due to its anti-bacterial properties. This was also one of the regimes of the Great Queens, Nefertiti and Cleopatra. These two were considered the most beautiful women ever. However, Nefertiti was thought to surpass Cleopatra with her beauty. Queen Esther also won the King's heart with her beauty regimes.   When using honey, make it RAW UN Purified honey! Benefits of raw honey for skin disorders and other ailments can be attributed to its antibiotic, anti-fungal, antiseptic and antibacterial properties.   Purified honey has very little healing properties due to destruction of nutrients during heating and pasteurization. It is known to increase production of collagen fibers and improving skin elasticity.

Then about once every two weeks, I mash a 1/4 of an avocado. Yes, a real edible avocado. I mash this and then put on my face as a mask. Leave it sitting for 15 to 30 minutes. The mask dries and hardens to a clay like mask.   Ahh, the feeling after washing it off. Avocado is very high in antioxidants. Antioxidants can help neutralize free radicals and eliminate toxins from your body which are nefarious for the skin. Hence, regular intake of avocado or avocado oil will prove beneficial for a healthy, radiant and supple skin.

Then once on the alternating weeks, I make my amazing chocolate & phresh greens mask. Hey, I say, if you can't eat it! High anti-oxidants and energy power for your face, this is it! This is by far the most yummy mask of them all! Talk about Just mix 2 table spoons of RAW cocoa powder & 1 table spoons pHresh greens with purified water. Enough to make a yogurt like consistency or thicker. Spread on face just like any other mask and leave on 15 - 20 minutes. Your skin in the largest absorbing organ. The greens really penetrate the skin and the anti-oxidants of the cacao help fight free radicals. So Enjoy~! Nothing like a chocolaty smell and licking your lips clean kind of treatment!.   I call this the PHresh Chocolate Mask!   Hey, you get your greens and chocolate in one place!

Remember, there are many ways to be creative. This mask really does rejuvenate the skin and deep on a cellular level.

For those occasional blemishes, use tea tree oil to dot them about 3 times per day. Tea tree oil is an amazing remedy for blemishes, cuts, scrapes and even cold sores.

You will notice, if you follow my post on face book and twitter, that I experiment with different foods to use as mask. This keeps things fun and interesting. :-D I use bentonite clay as well for a face mask. This mask is great for metal detoxification and purifying of the skin.   It also makes a great body mask for reducing the appearance of cellulite. This clay is an ancient Indian remedy for many ailments. It is awesome for brushing teeth to whiten them. I simply mix the clay with baking soda and real salt for my tooth powder. Also, if you have a tooth ache or an abscess, then if you make a clay ball and put it on the tooth, mash it tightly on the tooth and sleep in it, cause it taste funky. When you awaken, you will notice a heavy metal taste in your mouth. Don't worry, it was the clay attracting all the heavy metals out of your infected area. Then simply spit the clay and brush your teeth as normal. There are so many things you can enhance your beauty with right out of your kitchen pantry.

The Joys of an EDIBLE Shower~

Ahhhh~ Nothing like an edible shower. Try this. Mix 3 tbl. honey w/1 Tbl. Coconut Oil. Then different bowl: mix 1 C. Turbinado sugar, 1/4 C. Avacado Oil, 1/4 C. Grapeseed Oil, a few drops essential oil of peppermint, or lemon/lime zest. Have on hand, crushed adzuki beans, your coconut oil, sea clay based soap and aloe vera plant. A different day mix: 1 C. Celtic Sea Salt or Phresh Himalayan Salt with 1/2 C. Hemp oil and add some lime juice and lime zest (peel). Great detoxifying scrub!

Before showering: Do a complete body DRY Brushing. Using an all natural hair brush, start from your toes and brush firmly and UP-wards toward your lymph nodes. Brush entire feet and legs working all the way up to your chest and lymph nodes. Brushing firmly to release toxins out through lymph. When you reach chest and neck areas brush down toward lymph nodes and heart area. Then raise your arms one at a time, now brush firmly down from your finger tips to your arm pits. This entire process should only take 3 minutes. Next get in a steamy HOT shower, rinse your entire body and hair. Using your aloe vera plant, wash your hair to rid any build up. Now wash your face with your sea clay soap and adzuki scrub.Rinse. Next, put your honey/coconut oil mix on your hair. Massage very well into scalp and working down to the ends. Massage head for at least 1 minute. Now use the remaining honey/coconut oil mix to massage into your face and neck. Leave mix on hair and face as you finish your shower. Don't worry about it running down, just lick your lips~! Yumm. Next you can use your sea clay soap or honey oatmeal soap to wash your entire body. Now your are ready to exfolliate. Use your sugar scrub and scrub your entire body. Working in circular massaging motions to allow your body to readily absorb your oils. Massage slowly being sure to exfoliate all parts of your awesome body, fingers, toes, feet, backs of hands , elbows and bum. Then don't forget to use your pumice/volcano stone for smoothing the roughness of your feet and toes and maybe palm of hands. Using a wide tooth comb, you are ready to comb through your honey hair making it silky and yummy.   OK, ready to rinse from head to toe, rinsing your hair well while massaging scalp. After shower, PAT dry only, so not to rub off your sheen/oils.   Next, use your Aloe Vera plant to massage the gel into your face, neck and where ever else you want a lift. You should also use some of the

Aloe Vera Plant Gel to massage into your hair for nutrients and a great healthy shine. Now you are ready to endulge in Cocoa Butter or Coconut Oil all over your entire body and face! Now that's what I call an 'EDIBLE' shower.   OH the joys! Your skin will thank you. Doing this 2 or 3 times per week, you will see the benefits and become lost if you don't do it. Enjoy~

**Remember, you can experiment with your own kitchen staples. Try using the zest of a lemon, lime or orange for your scrubs. Use apple cider vinegar for a hair treatment, just pour over entire head after shampoo and let set for 10 to 15 minutes for a stronger hair follicle and deep conditioning. The use of turbinado sugar is just a suggestion as it tends to be a little less expensive.

It is VERY important to nourish your body from the INSIDE to reflect that healthy radiance glow or shiny hair on the outside. There are NO quick fixes and if you do all I say here on this page but you do NOT EAT CLEAN, then you are only putting a 'mask / or band aid' on the real problem. However, this that I tell you here, will definitely nourish your skin and hair as these are all good edible nutrients that are absorbed through your LARGEST organ. What goes on your skin goes in your body, and vice versa...what goes in your body reflects on the outer shell of your body. I eat lots of fats, such as avocados, coconut oil, hemp oil and hemp seeds. I also enduldge in lots of dark RAW cacao powder for my smoothies and sweet treats. Then I have to have my dark chocolate bar each day as well. Dark chocolate is so yummy and actually good for your skin. Make it organic and as dark as you can! Yes, RAW dark cacao NOT (cocoa) is high in anti-oxidants and nutrients. So EAT it and WEAR it! You really ARE what you eat. My friend Shan Stratton, of Core Health Products, says "You are what you absorb". Please also take care when choosing that right supplement. Also take care and caution with your food choices. Avoid chemical laden and processed foods as well as all the artificial crap they push down your throats. Make it REAL and WHOLE food and Organic supplements. A good digest enzyme is the key to proper nutrition and digestion. We could have this with food ONLY, however with the centuries of soil depletion, it is nearly impossible for even the best of organic food to properly help us digest our foods. Therefore we DO need that proper enzyme to help our body ecology. Also, please do not forget to eat many greens each day such as kale, broccoli, spinach, spirulina, barley, wheat grass and etc. If you just cannot seem to eat this many greens in one day, then I encourage you to check out my trusted 'on the go' friend, PHresh Greens! These super living greens are amazing. All you need is 1, yes ONE teaspoon mixed in water or juice or a smoothie per day. This amount of will give you your complete daily intake of greens. Perfect for travels! I do preach everything I practice myself. I do NOT eat GMO's, I avoid MSG's and eat as clean as I possibly can. If I must go out to eat, I find an organic restaurant or find a trusted sushi restaurant.

I NOURISH my body and skin from WITH IN~!

Also make sure you get plenty of daily exercise, and enough exercise to 'sweat' out the toxins that clog your pores. Yoga, pilates and a simple cardio routine at least 3 times per week will be sufficient. If you can't exercise enough to sweat, then please try incorporating a Far Infrared Sauna to help you 'sweat it out'. You can obtain one of these beauties for less than $2500.00 from Great Saunas. Or if you do not want to purchase a sauna, then check out your town for spa who offers these far infrared saunas on a daily use basis. You have always heard, "get your beauty rest". This is so very true...sleep your way to beauty. Sleep plays an important role in activating our cells to work properly. It is only during hours of deep sleep that our bodies are reset to run smoothly the next day. Our cells can only properly repair themselves during our sleeping life. More about sleep in future books. So be sure to watch for that. Get your zzzz's, at least 8 hours of sleep each and every night. You may also want to set one night a week to count your 'blessings' early. Try going to bed at least by 8:30 one time per week every week and waking at your normal time, 6a.m. or 7. Again, there is NO magic wand to wave to throw beauty your way. YOU ARE BEAUTIFUL, you just need to nurture your inner beauty to let it radiate on the outside!

You can basically find all your skin care needs in your kitchen pantry. Try experimenting with making your own sugar & salt scrubs. You want to have that healthy glow for the rest of your body as well as your face. Try mixing 1 cup of Turbinado sugar with 3/4 C. Avocado, Sunflower, or Grape seed or Olive oil. Add some rosemary or lemon or orange zest and even mix a Tbl. Honey with it. Use daily in shower for that soft skin feel and look! Then try mixing 1 cup Celtic Sea Salt or PHresh Himalayan Salt with same oils as the sugar scrub for a really invigorating feel and buffer for your skin. Plus you are absorbing the awesome minerals from the salt for that healthy glow! Then try adding Essential Oil of Myrr, or Primrose oil or even Peppermint for that stimulating effect. Myrr is so romantic! There are so many options and INEXPENSIVE choices right in your kitchen or garden! Please make kitchen staples ORGANIC.

So you see, my routine is very basic and very edible, and yummy!

You can do this. You are beautiful. You are amazing. You are LOVED!

Ok, so there you have your first introduction to eating and living a healthier lifestyle. There is so much more I could tell you right now and I so want to, but this is just the first step to get you on your way to cleaning up your food. I hope you found this to be enlightening as well as beneficial to your health. I encourage you to call if you should have any questions or email me. I challenge you to always keep these staples in your pantry.

Read all the way to the end for helpful sites and more information on how to live a vibrant radiant life.

Please stay tuned for the up and coming additions to this book. Book 2 goes into more detail about the different foods and how far the food industry has gotten off track. Book 3 is geared to my Christian friends as to why we should be eating the way I suggest. These are books filled with more enlightening information you will not want to miss out on.

Everything I mention in my book is *'Organic Guru' Approved*. All the listings in the back pages here are intended to be read as well and know WHO I support. Although there are many trusted companies I trust out there, I only have limited time and space to post them here. Check out my web page frequently for blogs, new companies and my recommendations.

LIVE HAPPY. BE PURE!

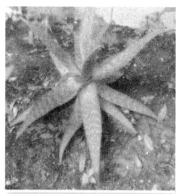

Aloe Vera Plant

Mucopolysaccharides +
Flavonoid antioxidants

~Fights free radicals
~Relieves dry skin
~Burn remedy
~Anti-Aging properties
~Improves Collagen
~Anti-Inflamatory
~Anti-Bacterial

One of Lynnette's skin care
home treatments. The beloved
age defying ALOE PLANT!
Simply saturate face and neck
with this gel and rest with it
overnight to wake up refreshed!
Used since B.C. with Cleopatra
and Nefertiti. LOVE the skin
you're IN. Nourish with CARE
and REAL earth!
More tips at: fuelforthebody.org

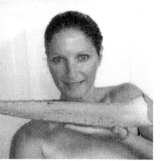

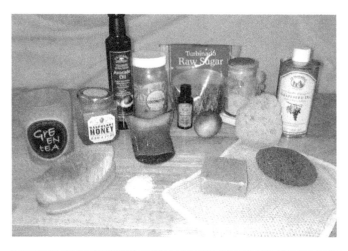

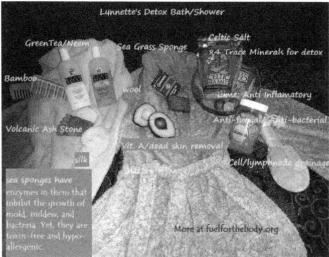

Please also keep in mind that all products I mention in here are what I use. By all means, if you have a company you love, then please use that company. The goal is to have many companies to be pure.

Also, I like using visuals for my audience to relate to. Most of my clients do not know where to start or what the item would even look like. So I use these companies to give visual. Although these companies are very pure. I do not have a store that I sell them in either. Now, you can go on my website and order at a discount, but I rarely do that as I encourage you to go shop and support your local health food store or grocery store that carry great organic products. Please do not think that I am trying to sell you on one thing or company. I do not, these are only examples and my personal choices.

Healthy SECRETS for Abundant Life

Here are a few Healthy tips from me to get you started on your way to a life full of health and longevity.

1.   First and foremost, CHANGE your food! Avoid processed foods, preserved foods or color additives & refined sugars & salts. Be Toxic FREE!

2.   Read Fuel for the Body...the Pate Weigh 'and follow the protocol.

3.   Know the truth about salt. Eat pure salt such as Celtic Sea Salt or Himalayan salt. Know the truth about sugar and all those "fake" sweeteners. Read article below.

4.   Avoid GMO = genetically modified organisms. Also avoid MSG = monosodium glutamate.

5.   Buy or grow ONLY all Organic & natural foods.

6.   Get rid of microwaves: they kill all living enzymes.

7.   Get a water filter for drinking and bathing. One that removes ALL fluoride and chlorine.

8.   Incorporate a 55 – 85% RAW food diet. Preferably 85% to reap the most beneficial enzymes that food has to offer.

9.   If you are a meat eater, look for local farmers whom raise AND harvest animals humanely and are fed an all-natural diet.

10.   When considering skin-care, remember, your skin is your largest organ. It absorbs the toxins to the blood stream. Buy or make all organic products.

11.   Eat HEMP every day! Eat extra virgin coconut oil every day! (use it for skin care too!) Drink apple cider vinegar every day! (diluted w/water of course)

12.   Get daily vitamin D from nature's SUN...it's FREE!

13.   Incorporate exercise every day. Try a rebounder, one that is strong and is made to give maximum benefits. Try a "cellerciser".

14.   Get a Far Infrared Sauna for your own personal use. Daily sauna use enhances sweat activity therefore eliminating toxins.

15.   Get daily intake of Purified Oxygen therapy. AKA: Oxygen Bars. You can purchase smaller units for personal home use. These are great for fighting cancer cells, bacteria and free radicals.

16.   Concentrate on daily laughter! Look for Laughter Yoga classes, these are a great way to get your laughter ignited. Laughter releases endorphins to help defray illnesses.

17.   Get regular Chiropractic adjustments to help the central nervous system. Regular adjustments also help to move lactic acid build up.

18.   Get deep tissue massages. These are great for relieving toxin build up on the muscles.

19.   Do FRESH juicing daily. Try a juice fast for at least 3 days! If you can't seem to get your greens in and juice, then incorporate pHresh Greens daily.

20.   Laugh, Hug & Pray every day!

LIVE HAPPY. BE PURE!

Last but certainly not least, I want to stress to you the importance of supporting your local and organic farmers. Demand to know what is in your food supply. Help us take a stand against our evil food empire, Monsanto. Do you really know what you are feeding your family? Do you really know what genetics lurk in your family's meals? The truth of the matter is that our food supply is getting stricken by the infestations of the toxic chemicals and the genetically modifying of organisms that Monsanto is force feeding us. We demand the right to choose what foods we eat and what supplements we give our families.

Please follow our bicycle T.O.U.R.s across the nation as we reach out to get our FDA to listen to our NO and say NO to Monsanto. We take your voices to stand UP for our food & health FREEDOMS!

Want health care reform? Then reform your kitchen pantry and invest in YOU!

My favorite saying: *"The problem is not the problem, the problem is your attitude about the problem".* *Captain Jack Sparrow.* This is so true. How will you handle your problems?

Healthful Information Sites

All information on companies and sites I mention throughout my book and the pages to follow are *ORGANIC GURU RECOMMENDED*! We practice the LIVE HAPPY. BE PURE! Life style.

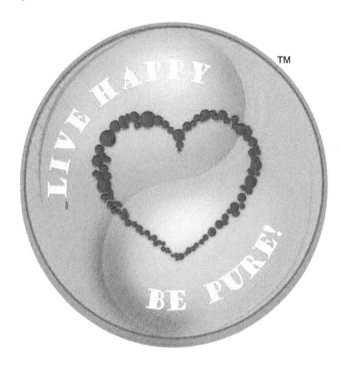

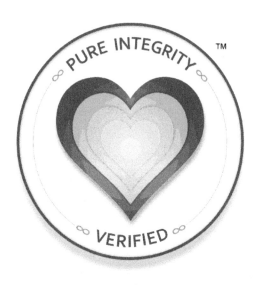

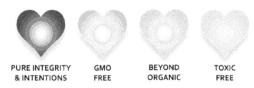

| PURE INTEGRITY & INTENTIONS | GMO FREE | BEYOND ORGANIC | TOXIC FREE |

Want to know what companies are practicing the pure and toxic free virtues? The above seal IS the seal of all the world households.   Please read more below.

MISSION STATEMENT

Pure Integrity Verified™ Seal of Approval brings to the world one of the highest quality standards in the industry. The Pure Integrity Verified™ seal of approval, is the household name for organic products so you don't have to worry about your purchases. Only the purest of products on the planet will gain PIV seal of approval. Helping the world to know about GMO's as well as the toxic chemicals that are being sprayed on our planet. Reflecting non-compromising standards so that you may be assured of PURE INTEGRITY products to bring in your home. Helping the world to understand the importance of knowing their food sources and getting to know their farmers. Dedicating timeless efforts to assure you and your children of a safe and toxic free future.

LIVE HAPPY. BE PURE!

VISION

Pure Integrity Verified™ Seal of Approval's vision is to help heal the world with purity and a quality life style. By setting the standards for Pure Integrity, there is no room for compromise or for sickness and diseases. Living a quality life style can be obtained and will help heal the world. Continually touring the world to enlighten the public of the importance of real foods and a chemical free planet will help us all to continue to make a difference TOGETHER. Engaging in relationships are the start of healing the planet. Visiting farms world-wide, we will help you get acquainted with local farmers in your area. A sick nation will surely fall but a healthy nation will conquer ALL! Together We Will Make a Difference~

www.vanishingbees.com
Honeybees have been mysteriously disappearing across the planet, literally vanishing from their hives. Known as Colony Collapse Disorder, this phenomenon has brought beekeepers to crisis in an industry responsible for

producing apples, broccoli, watermelon, onions, cherries and a hundred other fruits and vegetables. Commercial honeybee operations pollinate crops that make up one out of every three bites   of   food   on   our   tables. The film explores the struggles that bee keepers face as the two friends plead their case on Capitol Hill and travel across the Pacific Ocean in the quest to protect their honeybees.

Filming across the US, in Europe, Australia and Asia, this documentary examines the alarming disappearance of honeybees and the greater meaning it holds about the relationship between mankind and mother earth. As scientists puzzle over the cause, organic beekeepers indicate alternative reasons for this tragic loss. Conflicting options abound and after years of research, a definitive answer has not been found to this harrowing mystery.

www.organicconsumers.org   This site will help you navigate all your organic needs. They even have browsers set for you to find local organic coops and farmer's markets in your area. Here, you can find the latest news on farms, big corporations and much more insight to organic farming and supplies.

www.cheftinajo.com   You don't have to be 100% raw to get the benefits of nature's diet. I believe that if you maintain a 75% raw vegan lifestyle, you will look and feel amazing. But that doesn't mean you can scarf on burgers and cheese fries the other 25% of the time! Not all cooked food is created equal. If being 100% raw isn't for you, be sure to choose healthy cooked foods the rest of the time.

Hippocrates said "Let thy food be thy medicine", and it is so true! Cooked foods create disease-causing free radicals, while live raw vegan foods provide an abundance of disease-fighting antioxidants directly to your cells. A lot of folks report significant improvements with a variety of health issues upon transitioning to a high percentage of raw vegan foods. If you've read my bio, you know that I'm one of them.

www.selinanaturally.com

This site will give you access to the best of organic and 'real' products on the market. They pride themselves in optimum health!

Selina Naturally® connects people with products and information to empower mindful choices toward a healthier life. We also endeavor to introduce customers to uncommon artisan products from around the globe that are unique both in the benefits they impart and the opportunities they create. We focus on whole foods-based nutrition, supporting individuals through every step of their journey toward improved health.

Selina Naturally®, home of Celtic Sea Salt® brand.

www.bragg.com

Check this website out for amazing health stories and the story about the Founder, Paul Bragg. Also check out the story of Jack Lalane who is still alive and thriving and fit at the ripe young age of 97!

Paul, and his daughter, Patricia, have been health pioneers for decades. When the 'engineered fast food' products of science and industry had captured the attention of most Americans, Paul Bragg campaigned for a diet and lifestyle that focused on natural live foods and a healthy regime for a vital and long life. These ideas, based around natural and organic foods, are gaining praise and acceptance world-wide.

The Bragg Healthy Lifestyle Motto: "You are what you eat, drink, breathe, think, say and do".

www.greatsaunas.com

I mention using a sauna in my 20 tips to a vibrant, radiant and healthy life. Imagine, taking care of some of your health needs right in the comfort of your own home!

DETOXIFICATION

Since the skin is our largest organ, it plays an important role in eliminating undesirable toxins. Some physicians refer to the skin as a third kidney. The deep penetration of our West Coast Saunas' infrared technology allows removal of toxins stored in fat cells. Detoxifying in a West Coast Sauna helps rid your body of potential carcinogenic heavy metals such as mercury and lead, as well as alcohol, nicotine, sodium, sulfuric acid and cholesterol.

WEIGHT LOSS

As you bask in the comforts of a *Great Sauna*, your body is actually hard at work attempting to maintain a constant core temperature. Our body does this by increasing peripheral blood flow and by sweating. In Guyton's textbook of Medical Physiology, it states that 1 gram of sweat requires 0.568 kcal to produce. An average sauna user can produce 500 grams of sweat and burn 350 calories during a therapeutic sauna session. This is the equivalent of running 2-3 miles. Our infrared saunas can also help rid your body of cellulite which is a gel like substance made up of fat cells, water and wastes. *FEEL THOSE EXTRA POUNDS MELT AWAY!*

www.cellerciser.com

Why Cellercise® . . . There are many forms of exercise and most work the body as individual muscles or muscle groups. Since there are so many areas of the body to target, a typical exercise program can take up a lot of time. In addition a majority of exercises tear down to build up. The accumulative affect over time can be very damaging. Cellercise is the ultimate exercise as it flexes all 75 trillion cells at the same time! Even better, it requires only 10 minutes a day! By using vertical movement like weight lifting, push-ups, pulls-ups or sit-ups in a repetitive up and down motion against gravity, Cellercise targets ALL areas of the body at the same time.

www.nikken.com/prosperity4u
PiMag® Aqua Pour® Gravity Water System

Using an ingenious gravity flow system, the PiMag® Aqua Pour® Gravity Water System can provide you with Nikken PiMag® water no matter where you are. The Aqua Pour includes several stages of filtration, including a bed of mineral stones like those in streams and rivers. Pi ceramics are in the filter, to impart "the water of life." Nikken Magnetic Technology completes the process. The PiMag® Aqua Pour® is the most convenient way to set up a supply of PiMag® water practically anywhere.

www.seedtimetoharvest.com
Organic Pro Gardener, Joy Scroggie will enlighten you on the exciting avenues of growing your own abundance of real wholesome foods.

"Organic Food verses Commercial Food and the critical importance of getting away from a chemical life style"

Chemicals are killing us - they leave heavy metals & toxins in our bodies.

www.drleonardcoldwell.com
Dr. Leonard Coldwell: "I will not start the fight, but I will finish it!"

Dr. Leonard Coldwell is the world's leading authority for Cancer cures, Stress-Related Illness, and Burnout Syndrome, and is the most successful motivational and success trainer of our time.

He is the author of 19 bestselling books including his mega best sellers: The Only Answer to Cancer, and The Only Answer to Surviving Your Illness and Your Doctor. Over 57 million readers enjoy his teachings. His IBMS Stress Reduction CD set is the most endorsed and most sold of all times. Dr. Coldwell is the most endorsed and integrated natural Doctor in the world, having earned 4 doctor degrees and 4 PHDs. He recently received an honorary doctor degree in Humanity from the University in Louisiana for his achievements for cancer patients and for the improvement of quality of life for humans.

www.theearthdiet.com
Liana Werner-Gray is considered an Expert in Health and Nutrition and through The Earth Diet has guided people with the following...   · To Lose Weight/ Gain Weight/ Gain Muscle/ MuscleTone/ Restore the body to natural weight /Rid cellulite
· To treat and reverse ALL dis-ease including anything "incurable", diabetes, cancer, skin disorders, arthritis and more
· To treat additions, food and eating disorders
· To assist people to detox/cleanse the body and boost the Immune System
· To Educate in RAW food making and getting the most nutrition out of foods!
· To live a harmonious life in balance with the Human Body and Organic Seasonal Nature. More inside the book!

www.phreshproducts.org

Our Mission:

Our mission is to be the premier authority regarding   pH balance in all aspects of our living environment. We strive to reflect the highest ethical standards in all product production and development while informing the global community on the importance of "Maintaining Health...Not Sickness". We strive to be the leading global innovator, developer of all types of pH products available.   With this effort, we bring a greater understanding to the Global community of the importance of health, wellness and balance in our daily lives.

Our Vision

Maintain Health ... Not Sickness. That's what it's all about. It's the reason why we are committed to inspire well-being (from the inside out). We strive for SMILES. We profit from POSITIVITY. We hold our HEALTH and HAPPINESS in our

HEARTS. We are a TEAM. We are a FAMILY. We are more than a business, we are a COMMUNITY! At Personal Health Product Development, we are steadfast in our mission to change the world through proper education and nutrition. We create our products with true intention, focusing on preventative care and wellness. You, our people, our customers, our team, are our shareholders. You help us to help the world by lending your support and spreading the love .

We thank you greatly for your support in us and in our mission.

**If you follow me on social media and in the news, you will see that I am one of pHresh Products' Super Stars. Together we work to get the world to "Maintain Health and NOT Sickness'.

A HUGE THANK YOU TO OUR SPONSORS~

Please take a look at the wonderful contributing sponsors' ads in the pages to follow. Our sponsors have been very instrumental in helping my Fuel for the Body Bike Team achieve the goal of pedaling thousands of miles across the nation and around the world to educate and empower the public about organic and natural living as well as saying NO to Monsanto and the Food Industry. Please follow us on face book at: www.facebook.com/fuelforthebody to find out more detailed information of the amazing T.O.U.R. There you will find how to be a part of our team, how to have your voice heard and how to sponsor this great cause on our next tour. More information also at www.fuelforthebody.org

I have provided you with great resources in this book to help you help your selves and help you have access to some wonderful companies. I invite you to use these resources to help you live a vibrant, radiant and healthful lifestyle.

Always: LIVE HAPPY. BE PURE!

Namaste~

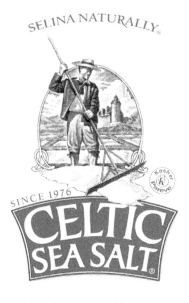

Celtic Sea Salt® is a Nutritious
Sea Salt with Vital Trace Minerals
1.800.TOP.SALT

www.celticseasalt.com

www.SelinaNaturally.com

Selina Naturally™ connects people with products and
information to empower mind-full choices toward a healthier
lifestyle.

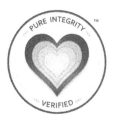

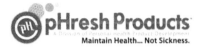

Our Mission:

Our mission is to be the premier authority regarding   pH balance in all aspects of our living environment. We strive to reflect the highest ethical standards in all product production and development while informing the global community on the importance of "Maintaining Health...Not Sickness". We strive to be the leading global innovator, developer of all types of pH products available.   With this effort, we bring a greater understanding to the Global community of the importance of health, wellness and balance in our daily lives.

www.phreshproducts.com

4023 Kennett Pike, Suite 622
Greenville, DE 19807

(888) 901-6150 support@phreshproducts.com

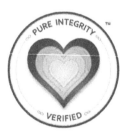

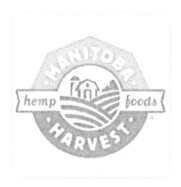

www.manitobaharvest.com
1-800-665-HEMP(4367)   Canada

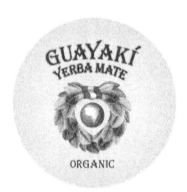

www.guayaki.com

We are an organization of individuals who's daily work is to bring you the finest yerba mate on the planet. We started 1996 with a vision of protecting and restoring the South American rainforests and empowering the native forest people, and with your help, we are achieving that goal, sip by sip.

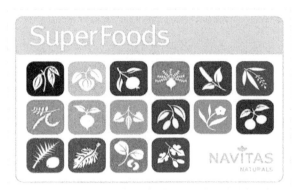

www.navitasnaturals.com

(888) 645-4282

The "Navitas" in our name is the Latin word for energy. And like our name implies, our mission is to provide premium organic functional foods that increase energy and enhance health. Navitas Naturals is a certified organic, green business headquartered in Marin County, California. We specialize in organic and wild-crafted functional foods, and strive to lead the industry in this expanding market.

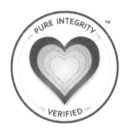

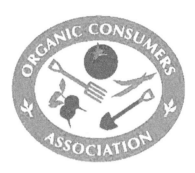

The Organic Consumers Association (OCA) is an online and grassroots non-profit 501(c)3 public interest organization campaigning for health, justice, and sustainability. The OCA deals with crucial issues of food safety, industrial agriculture, genetic engineering, children's health, corporate accountability, Fair Trade, environmental sustainability and other key topics. We are the only organization in the US focused exclusively on promoting the views and interests of the nation's estimated 50 million organic and socially responsible consume.
www.organicconsumers.org

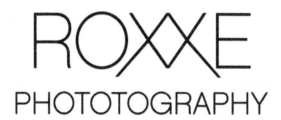

www.roxxephotography.com

ECCO BELLA

Ecco Bella was started to provide cruelty free organic cosmetics and natural skin care products. Free of Anything You Won't Like! NO water, gluten, dyes or preservatives. Besides speaking out for animals and the environment, our products help you conserve money. Why? Each Ecco Bella product multi-tasks. For example, all the skin care products are so rich in beneficial ingredients they claim both anti-aging and anti-blemish benefits combined! That means fewer products to buy, and they really work!

www.eccobella.com   877- 696-2220

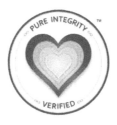

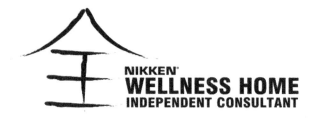

www.nikken.com/prosperity4u

The Nikken vision includes an understanding that total wellness rests on the 5 Pillars of Health. Healthy Body, Mind, Family, Society and Finances. Balance in all of these areas can help produce a more healthy and satisfying lifestyle.

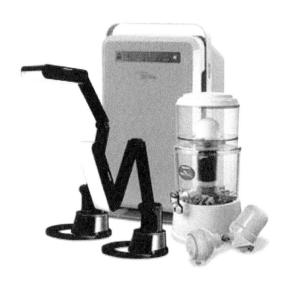

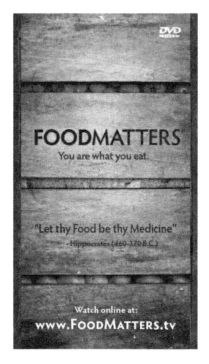

With nutritionally-depleted foods, chemical additives and our tendency to rely upon pharmaceutical drugs to treat what's wrong with our malnourished bodies, it's no wonder that modern society is getting sicker. Food Matters sets about uncovering the trillion dollar worldwide 'sickness industry' and gives people some scientifically verifiable solutions for overcoming illness naturally.

www.foodmatters.tv

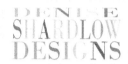 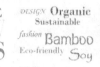

Welcome to Denise Shardlow Designs.

We are a sustainable business committed to creating clothing that fits easily into your lifestyle. Our collections are versatile, timeless, wonderfully wearable and created with a low environmental footprint.   Denise Shardlow is Lynnette's personal designer.

www.shardlowdesigns.com

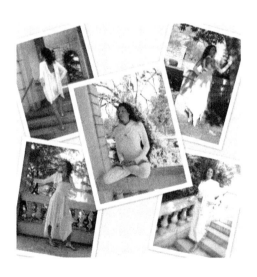

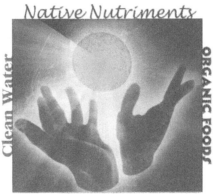

Healing Body Mind and Spirit

www.nativenutriments.com

Our oils come from around the world from the highest of quality plants and herbs we can find. Wild crafted and beyond organic and practices the integrity of fair trading. They treat those that come with emotional, physical, and spiritual concerns. For those that cannot come to our healing center, we have this site so you can gift and be gifted with our Essential oils, our bedding, and our immune herbs and whole food vitamins.

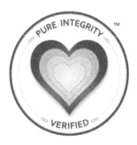

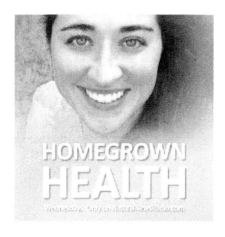

With Joni Abbott

www.naturalnewsradio.com

My Personal Trainer, Donovan Green, as well as Dr.
Oz Personal Trainer

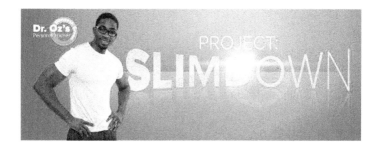

www.projectslimdown.com

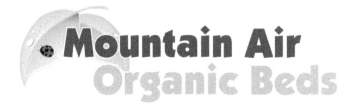

www.mountainairorganicbeds.com

Not only is it important to eat organic and drink organic, but equally important to sleep organic. We spend one third of our lives in the bed. Think about that for a moment. Made of latex from the sustainable rubber tree plants. Never wears out!

Could your health be at risk?

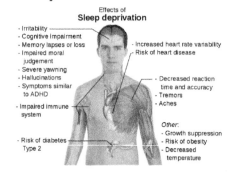

Effects of
Sleep deprivation

- Irritability
- Cognitive impairment
- Memory lapses or loss
- Impaired moral judgement
- Severe yawning
- Hallucinations
- Symptoms similar to ADHD
- Impaired immune system
- Risk of diabetes Type 2

- Increased heart rate variability
- Risk of heart disease
- Decreased reaction time and accuracy
- Tremors
- Aches

Other:
- Growth suppression
- Risk of obesity
- Decreased temperature

It doesn't matter if you spend $300 or $3,000 on a regular mattress. It's going to break down in 5 -7 years and Sleeping on a broken mattress causes pain!

Mountain Air
Organic Beds
Bigger, Better, Stronger and More Healthful ™

Order & learn more here:
mountainairorganicbeds.com

236

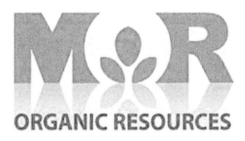

ORGANIC RESOURCES

MōR® Organic Resources strives to offer the best raw and organic products available

Moringa is on the same market segment as "green superfoods" such as spirulina, green barley, wheat and alfalfa sprouts. It is also similar in composition and effects as Noni juice, also called Morinda citrifolia.

Modern research has found that Moringa leaves, as well as other parts of the tree, have been used since ancient times as traditional ayurvedic medicine in several cultures such as a natural antibiotic, an aid in childbirth, for treating liver disorders and many other uses. Moringa has been used for inflammation, malnutrition, wounds, diabetes, iron deficiency, high blood pressure and other conditions.

Containing over 90 nutrients and 46 antioxidants, Moringa (Moringa Oleifera) is one of nature's most nutritious foods. Ideal for helping our bodies maintain optimum health. Moringa leaves are highly nutritious and are rich in vitamins K, A, C, B6, Manganese, Magnesium, Riboflavin, Calcium, Thiamin, Potassium, Iron, Protein and Niacin

www.organic-moringa.com

ORGANIZATIONS I SUPPORT

The organizations that are listed here in the next few pages are near and dear to my heart. I encourage you to check out these amazing organizations who are steadily working to make our world a healthy and happy world!

We have yearly events in which to help raise funds for these organizations. We also donate portions of proceeds from sales that are made through our different outlets in stores or online.

American Anti-Cancer Institute: a wellness facility that is in the process of being built in Washington state. Founded by Robert Wright, Author of Killing Cancer NOT People. With his organization and board members, they help people with cancer to reverse their disease. If you are in need of phone consultations, Bob is available via phone and can help you along your journey.

The Mission of the proposed American Anti-Cancer Center Campus, is to eradicate cancer and other immune-degenerative disease in humans through the Hippocratic philosophy of Natural Medicine among three proposed Campus facilities: The American Anti-Cancer Institute, The American Anti-Cancer University and The American Anti-Cancer Clinic.

Vision and Philosophy: By re-educating the public, our Vision is for a new day to dawn upon the United States in which cancer is understood to be a rare but curable disease of the immune system. (More here) We believe that the philosophy of conventional American healthcare (centered in pharmaceuticals, surgery—and in the case of cancer, radiation and chemotherapy) has failed to provide U.S. citizens with true health and lasting healing. As cancer rates rise to plague an estimated 50% of adult Americans by the end of 2012, we believe a massive paradigm shift in cancer care is the only way for Americans to regain our physical and economic strength. Our inspiration is American children for whom cancer is now the leading cause of death among all disease categories.

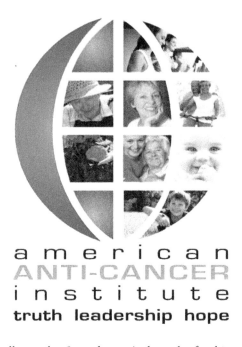

american
ANTI-CANCER
institute
truth leadership hope

You will note that I am also an Ambassador for this unique organization. We help to raise funds and awareness via our events and tours. Help us help save the life of a loved one.

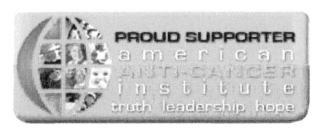

www.americanaci.org

Next is the Gerson Treatment center in Baja, Mexico. Dr. Patrick Vickers is the founder and facilitator of this life saving clinic. They help you to retrain your brain to have better eating habits. They have extensive retreats to help your body rid itself of diseases such as cancers, HPV, and many others. They also have an excellent protocol for completely getting the drug addict no longer addicted to drugs and start a clean slate. If you have someone with a life threatening disease or drug abuse or sickness they just cannot get over, then check out the Gerson hospital today.

Dr. Patrick Vickers helps me with my kidney ailments and stays abreast of my concerns along with my holistic kidney doctor, Jenna Henderson. Because of them, I am on my way to complete and constant healing.

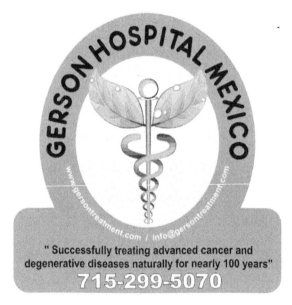

" Successfully treating advanced cancer and degenerative diseases naturally for nearly 100 years"
715-299-5070

Next is an amazing organization that helps save lives of children in 3rd world countries. These children and their families do not have the means to afford hospitals, much less afford surgeries that can save their child. These are children who would die without the surgery. Yes, we know that all diseases and ailments can be prevented and cured. However, when you have children who are sick and on a death bed, they are already toxic and simple diets cannot change their destiny. Therefore, surgeries are needed, then we teach them to eat a more healthy diet. See how YOU help us to save children's lives by simply making purchases of PHresh products on my site or in stores near you. See, we really are making differences in the world we live in. THANK YOU for purchasing Phresh Products. See the story of little Jaime's life- saving journey below.

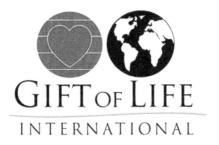

GIFT OF LIFE
INTERNATIONAL

www.giftoflifeinternational.org

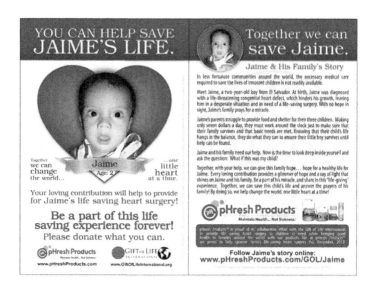

Your purchase of pHresh products helped a family keep their child alive! Now your purchase of this book, is helping to save another child's life and spare a family's heartache.

I am available for private consultations in person, via phone or skype. My assistants will help you set up your consult.   I will be your personal coach as well your cheerleader.   I listen and have compassion. You will have the tools you need to easily transition from the toxic world into the life of longevity.

I am also available for public seminars to educate and empower the public about organic and sustainable living.

Call today to schedule your consultation or book a seminar.

What is YOUR health worth to you? Invest in YOU. Let your food be your health insurance policy.

Lynnette Marie, your Organic Guru
Medicine Woman & Minister for the Environment

LIVE HAPPY. BE PURE!

www.fuelforthebody.org
getfueled@fuelforthebody.org
www.facebook.com/fuelforthebody
417-365-7805

***The statements in this book are not meant for treatment, cure or prevention of any disease or sickness and these statements have not been regulated by the FDA.

CPSIA information can be obtained at www.ICGtesting.com
Printed in the USA
LVOW05s0155280715

447861LV00029B/470/P